The Concise Guide to Homoeopathy

Nigel and Susan Garion-Hutchings are homoeopaths with many years of professional practice behind them. They have written this book from both professional and personal experience, as they not only run a successful practice in Brighton at their School for Developmental Studies and Holistic Therapies, but have also successfully raised a family of five boys using homoeopathy.

The Concise Guide to
Homoeopathy

An Introduction to
the Understanding and Use of
Homoeopathy

Nigel and Susan Garion-Hutchings

ELEMENT
Shaftesbury, Dorset • Rockport, Massachusetts
Brisbane, Queensland

First published in 1988
by the Wellbeing Foundation

This edition first published
in Great Britain in 1993 by
Element Books Limited
Longmead, Shaftesbury, Dorset

Published in the USA in 1993 by
Element, Inc
42 Broadway, Rockport, MA 01966

Published in Australia in 1993 by
Element Books Limited for
Jacaranda Wiley Limited
33 Park Road, Milton, Brisbane 4064

Cover illustration by Rosanne Sanders
Cover design by Max Fairbrother
Designed by Roger Lightfoot
Typeset by The Electronic Book Factory Ltd,
Fife, Scotland
Printed and bound in Great Britain by
Dotesios Ltd, Trowbridge, Wiltshire

British Library Cataloguing in Publication
data available

Library of Congress Cataloging in Publication
data available

ISBN 1–85230–384–0

Contents

Acknowledgements vi
How This Book is Laid Out vii
Introduction ix

Part One
1. The History of Homoeopathy 2
2. Laws and Principles of Homoeopathy 9
3. Homoeopathy – A Holistic Approach 16
4. Homoeopathic Philosophy 21
5. The Course of Dis-ease and the Return to Health 29

Part Two
6. The Work of the Homoeopathic Prescriber 36
7. Test Case Examples Using the Grid 42
8. Guidelines to Taking the Remedies 54

Part Three
9. The Remedy Pictures 58
Aconite 59 · *Apis mellifica* 62 · *Arsenicum album* 64
Belladonna 66 · *Bryonia* 68 · *Calcarea carbonica* 70
Carbo vegetabilis 72 · *Chamomilla* 74 · *Cina* 76
Dulcamara 78 · *Gelsemium* 80 · *Hepar sulph* 82
Ignatia 84 · *Lycopodium* 86 · *Nux vomica* 87
Pulsatilla 89 · *Rhus toxicodendron* 92 · *Spongia* 94
Sulphur 95

Part Four
10. The First Aid Remedies 100
11. Conclusion 107

Answers to Test Cases 110
Glossary 111
Further Reading 116
Useful Addresses 117
Courses and Classes 120
Pharmacies 122
Index 126

Acknowledgements

Special thanks to our family, friends and patients for all their support and encouragement.

As above, so below. We gratefully acknowledge the awakening consciousness and give thanks for that and all who have helped to make this book a reality.

Thank you

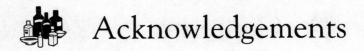

How this book is laid out

The Concise Guide to Homoeopathy is divided into four main parts.

Part One

Part One deals with the history, philosophy and principles on which homoeopathy is based. Read this section with care and consider the implications as there is much original thought here.

Part Two

Part Two summarizes some important aspects of Part One and leads into a full practical guide to case taking and prescribing in the true homoeopathic manner for the everyday acute ailments that one finds in every home from time to time. Many answers to the questions you will want to ask will be found in this section.

Some test cases are also provided in Part Two so that you may try your hand at finding the remedy. Also explained in this section is the easy to use symptom analysis grid which will help you to do this.

Part Three

Part Three is where the remedy pictures are described. This is a reference section which needs to be frequently referred to when looking for your remedy in any given case. How and why you need to do this is explained in Part Two.

Part Four

Part Four comprises the first aid remedies which are applied in a different way than the general remedies. These remedies and their method of application are described fully in this section.

An at-a-glance guide to the first aid remedies' sphere of usefulness can also be found in Part Four.

A glossary of terms that may be unfamiliar to the reader has been provided at the back of the book. To help your understanding, refer to it as required.

Also at the back of the book you will find the answers to the test cases in Part Two, and some useful addresses.

Introduction

In this guide we attempt, in a concise manner, to consider the history, philosophy and principles on which homoeopathy is based. From this the foundation is laid for those who wish to take their studies further.

We have also attempted to provide a concise guide which, when followed, will take you on a journey full of new and exciting discoveries; one of which is how to use homoeopathic remedies/medicines with safety, effectiveness and speed, for the everyday common ailments and complaints that can be found in every home from time to time.

This has been done without losing the essential element of homoeopathy which lies in its adaptability and depth of action. Homoeopathy in essence is a way of life, a new way of perceiving the world, which is rewarding and fulfilling.

Homoeopathy encourages a quality of life free from negative attitudes and emotions with their corresponding physical complaints. When used with understanding and depth of perception, homoeopathy can change the course of peoples' lives and encourage a quality of life which is unsurpassed.

This guide will set you on a road of adventures where you can take responsibility for being a positive contributor to this planet and the life it sustains.

The purpose of this book is to give you a glimpse of the world of homoeopathy in its most basic and practical aspect. The study of homoeopathy is fascinating and endless. One is always a student, in turn excited and delighted, as work, study and practice open yet more doors and reveal further truths and possibilities. For any newcomer to homoeopathy there are always the failures, accompanied by doubt, yet also there are many successes. The taste of this success, of getting it right, of seeing someone indisputably change from a state of sickness to a state of well-being after you have administered to them a little harmless homoeopathic pillule will stay with you forever. From that moment onwards you know by experience that it can and does work. You will realize what enormous possibilities exist to relieve suffering and change a direction from disharmony to harmony. And if, after this tiny glimpse and fleeting taste, you want to know and understand more you will surely not be disappointed. For this medical study goes far beyond medicine as we normally know it. There is always room to go further on, and the journey is as uplifting as the discoveries.

Wishing you an interesting, enjoyable and fruitful read.

Nigel and Susan Garion-Hutchings

Close your eyes and you will see clearly.
Cease to listen and you will hear truth.
Be silent and your heart will sing.
Seek no contacts and you will find union.
Be still and you will move forward on the tide of the spirit.
Be gentle and you will need no strength.
Be patient and you will achieve all things.
Be humble and you will remain entire.

Taoist Meditation

Part One

It is not believing in separateness but knowing that we are an integral part of all life.

1. The History of Homoeopathy

Samuel Hahnemann – the founder of homoeopathy

Samuel Hahnemann was born on 10th April 1755 in Meissen, one of the most beautiful parts of Germany. Hahnemann himself suggested that this may have contributed largely to his appreciation of the beauties of nature as he grew up to manhood. His father, Christian Gottfried Hahnemann, was a painter for the porcelain factory of the town. Samuel had great respect for his father and valued the advice and teachings that were passed on to him as to the conceptions of that which was good and could be called worthy of man. To act and live without pretence or show was his most noteworthy advice. Samuel was impressed more by his father's example than his words. His father, however, was not in favour of his son's keen desire to study and often kept him from school in order that he might pursue some business more suited to his income.

This did not deter the young Hahnemann who made it his duty to grasp what he was studying rather than study too much, to read little but correctly and to classify in his mind the portion already read before continuing. By the age of twelve, Samuel was teaching Greek to his fellow pupils in order to assist his father in the payment of the school fees. His teachers encouraged his inclination to study and prevented his father from interrupting his school work by refusing school fees during the last eight years.

In 1775 Samuel Hahnemann went to Leipzig with little money in his pocket and a burning desire to learn more. He was a gifted linguist and survived by teaching German and French to wealthy young Greeks. At the same time he translated medical books from English into German. This not only earned him his money but also supported his study.

Here at Leipzig University, Hahnemann studied privately and

attended the medical professors' lectures whenever he was able to get hold of a free lecture pass. He was to practise his father's maxim during these years – never to be a passive learner and by physical exercise and fresh air to encourage that energy and vigour which alone enable the body to stand successfully the strain of continued mental exertion.

At Leipzig Hahnemann became most discerning and only attended the lectures he considered to be the most useful. After two years of self study, attending lectures where possible, the young Hahnemann made his way to Vienna to study the practical side of medicine, for which there was no institution in Leipzig.

After only nine months he was forced to leave due to a malicious trick (he would not say what) that robbed him of all his savings. But the time had been spent well and Samuel Hahnemann had already acquired the friendship of Dr von Quarin, physician to the royal family. The doctor had allowed him to attend his private patients as an observer and spent much time encouraging and teaching his practical skills to the eager student.

Hahnemann's last crumbs of subsistence were just about to vanish when the Governor of Transylvania, Baron von Bruckenthal, invited him to go to Hermanstadt with him as his family physician and the custodian of his important library. Here he had the opportunity to learn several other languages and some sciences in which he felt lacking. He practised medicine here for twenty-one months before leaving to receive his medical degree at Erlaugen.

On 10th August 1779 Samuel Hahnemann received his degree of Doctor of Medicine. During the next two years he practised medicine, never for very long in one place, and added to his store of knowledge through more self study.

Towards the end of 1781 he was offered the post of Medical Officer of Health for Gommein, near Magdeburg. During the three years here Samuel married Henrietta, an apothecary's step-daughter. They moved to Dresden and spent four years there working in the hospitals before moving back to Leipzig in 1789 in order to be nearer the 'source of science', as Hahnemann put it. By this time Samuel and Henrietta's family had grown to four daughters and one son.

These years were very difficult for Samuel and he is to be admired for his undaunted courage, force of decision and strong will as much as for his modesty.

Hahnemann's disenchantment with medical science

It was during his years in Dresden that he recognized more fully the insufficiency of medical sciences and of the therapeutic methods of those days. With much energy and eloquence of speech he denounced the methods employed in the medical field.

From Dresden the Hahnemann family moved back to Leipzig. Here Samuel gave up the practice of medicine in favour of translating and other literary works in order to support his growing family.

During this period Hahnemann unreservedly fought the practice of bloodletting and purging. One incident in particular is worth a mention. In 1792 Kaiser Leopold XI of Austria died a sudden and painful death. The Kaiser was loved and respected for his insight and cleverness and had been able to preserve peace between France and Germany. France had threatened war against neighbouring Germany and everywhere hope was placed on Leopold's strategic intervention. In order to explain his sudden illness and death and so prevent wild rumours it was found necessary to explain the situation through a published bulletin issued by the physicians in charge.

In Hahnemann's attack on this bulletin, published in the *Anzeiger*, a popular paper of the time, he states:

> On the morning of 28th February his doctor, Langusius, found a severe fever and distended abdomen. He tried to fight the condition by venesection, and, as this failed to give relief, he repeated the process three times more, without any better result. We ask from a scientific point of view, according to what principles has anyone the right to order a second venesection when the first failed to bring relief? As for a third, heaven help us! But to draw blood a fourth time when the first three failed to alleviate! To abstract the fluid of life four times in 23 hours from a man who has lost flesh from mental overwork combined with a long continued diarrhoea without procuring any relief! Science pales before this!

Leopold died on 1st March, at 4.30pm whilst vomiting, in the presence of the Empress.

Hahnemann challenged the monarch's doctors to justify themselves publicly. This string of events naturally aroused great sensation, and long argument for and against Hahnemann raged in the *Anzeiger*.

A complete and accurate bulletin was promised from the monarch's physicians but this never appeared. Hahnemann, however, carried on the fight against bloodletting, purging and aperients with growing enthusiasm.

Hahnemann questions Dr Cullen's fever theory

Cullen's *Materia Medica* was also questioned specifically as to the medicinal effect of Peruvian bark, from which quinine is derived.

This marked the first milestone on the road to the development of a new method of treatment. Hahnemann vigorously opposed Cullen's idea that Peruvian bark proved effective in fevers due to its bitter properties and tonic effect on the stomach. To prove this point Hahnemann combined strong bitters and astrigents and pointed out that these combinations had more of both these properties than the bark, but could cure no fever. He went on to say that substances such as strong coffee, pepper, ignatia bean and arsenic produce intermittent fever and were also effective in counteracting them.

Dr Cullen was a much respected teacher of the time and so this attack by Hahnemann was regarded as highly controversial, similar to the effect any attack on the established medical practices would have today. This was seen in the reaction to Prince Charles' controversial speech to the BMA in 1982.

Hahnemann went on to experiment with the bark and reportedly took an ounce of the bark, and on the same day was attacked with 'cold fever' symptoms, similar to those of malaria. Hahnemann sensed that the effect a substance had on the healthy organism indicated its curative power for similar dis-ease symptoms.

It became clear at this point that Hahnemann had become

totally disillusioned with the medical practices of the time and the explanations given for their use by Cullen and others. He began to look in earnest for more reliable modes of treatment and clearer explanations for their use. For this purpose he began to experiment on himself by taking various medicinal substances and logging their results.

Hahnemann discovers the law of similars

From all his labours he deduced, partly by intuition and partly by logical reasoning, that substances that produced symptoms in a healthy human being could remove similar symptoms exhibited by a dis-eased individual. This became known as the law of similars.

At this time Samuel Hahnemann and his family were very poor and they were being hounded by the established medical fraternity. This state of affairs encouraged the benevolent Prince, Duke Ernest von Sachsen-Gotha, who was well acquainted with the learned man's plight, to step in and offer help. Hahnemann gratefully accepted and offered to treat Klockenbring, a distinguished gentleman who was mentally insane and known to the Duke. The Duke offered a wing of his hunting castle to Hahnemann for use as a nursing home.

Hahnemann again departed from the usual methods employed at that time which involved violent reprimands for all behaviour regarded as insane. He treated Klockenbring with love, firmness and respect. Diet was used judiciously as well as some remedies prepared by Hahnemann himself. All this resulted in a complete cure for Klockenbring, something previous physicians had failed to achieve.

Hahnemann laid stress on his metaphysical school system which Klockenbring had learned by listening to him. Even at this early stage, Hahnemann had abandoned the use of large quantities of drugs. Friendliness and humanity combined with firmness instil at the same time the necessary respect and confidence required for a cure. He abhorred the violence and brutality that was common in these cases at the time.

Samuel Hahnemann was a man of vision. He may have been regarded as eccentric at the time as he was not content to follow the accepted modes of treatment. This created antagonism and he was subjected to abuse from many established physicians.

Hahnemann was unable to maintain the nursing home and was once again rendered homeless. The cost of moving was extremely high and living in the town proved to be far too expensive. He only saved himself and his large family, now numbering ten, from ruin by fleeing to the country. The years following 1800 proved to be very difficult as Samuel was unable to practise his healing art due to his short stays in various provinces. Because of this he was unable to gain the confidence of the local inhabitants and was forced to support himself and his family primarily through his literary pursuits. Nevertheless, he continued his research and experiments during these difficult years.

His literary pursuits were hardly able to support his large family and so he was forced to accept patients and treat them by correspondence. This added to the attacks made upon him by his colleagues, as it was unheard of at the time. The attacks were continually repeated wherever he went, partly because of his success as a medical practitioner, and partly because he prepared his own medicines as he was a brilliant chemist.

Hahnemann was by no means afraid of stating his convictions and never shunned a fight which he thought was necessary. All of this must have put him and his family under considerable strain. When it affected his patients so they were afraid to visit him he would move on, only to be faced with the same trial elsewhere.

The Organon of medicine – Hahnemann's new mode of treatment

From the years 1790 to 1805 his new system of treatment was slowly coming to birth. By 1810 the *Organon* had been completed. The *Organon* contains Hahnemann's conception of the 'new' mode of treatment, stating clearly and precisely the principles and laws upon which homoeopathy rests.

Hahnemann, who was now completely opposed to the medical practices of the time, was forced to take refuge in hygiene and dietetics, whenever advising his patients. His advice during the late eighteenth and early nineteenth century revolved almost entirely around these approaches to health and few remedies were prescribed. He did however, indicate that diet was not to be universally applied and that one man's stomach was different from the next. He was also suggesting that cheerfulness and control of emotions were conducive to prevention of ill health. These concepts are generally thought today to be modern in approach, and certainly show Hahnemann's holistic attitude.

Hahnemann always took diet into account, in both acute and chronic illness, and until his old age it remained one of the methods of his curative treatment.

Next to food, Hahnemann propagated the idea that exercise was a most essential requirement for achieving and maintaining health. He felt that exercise and fresh air promoted good circulation, strengthened the heart and brought about healthy digestion.

His ideas did not really catch on until the 1950s and are only now beginning to catch the imagination of the general public. He was well ahead of his time in more ways than one.

2. Laws and Principles of Homoeopathy

The law of similars

The experiment that Hahnemann did with Peruvian bark revealed a law which was to become the foundation stone of homoeopathy. This law, *similia similibus curantur* (likes are to be cured with likes), was tried and tested in Hahnemann's time and is still being used today with ever-increasing success.

Hahnemann's idea was that two similar dis-eases could not exist in the body at the same time. That the stronger, similar dis-ease would displace the weaker. Hahnemann had observed this phenomenon when it occurred naturally. He believed that one should imitate nature, which at times heals a chronic dis-ease by another additional one.

Because the artificially produced dis-ease had no lasting power it did not stay around to cause long-time suffering. However, it would be successful in removing the original similar dis-ease, which would not return.

Prescribing according to the law of similars

In order to be able to prescribe according to the law of similars, we must realize that the symptoms which point towards the pathological condition of the patient and enable us to give it a diagnostic label are of least importance in deciding on the curative remedy. A patient may be described as having 'flu, or may be described by the name of the remedy which cures him. For example, an allopath may say this is a 'flu case', whereas a homoeopath may say 'this is a bryonia case', or whatever remedy was indicated by the individual's symptom picture. Ten people all exhibiting the common symptoms of 'flu may need ten different remedies according to their individual symptom pictures or, in other words, the way the individual is expressing and experiencing their dis-ease.

The provers and the remedy provings

Over the years, Hahnemann experimented extensively upon himself and his family and a growing band of followers. He instigated 'provings' by taking small doses of the drugs until a reaction was experienced. Every symptom produced would be carefully noted down – all symptoms being noted, whether they affected the mind, body or emotions. He also searched medical works for accounts of cures and poisonings. After a long period of study Hahnemann was confident that the new system of medicine, which he called *homoeopathy*, a Greek word meaning 'similar suffering', was true and consistent, and so he began to use it in clinical practice.

Potentization

However, he now encountered a new problem – dosage. He experimented with various strengths of the medicines because many of the substances used were highly toxic in their crude state and although diluting them reduced their side effects, it also, correspondingly decreased their curative powers. After much experimentation he came across another extremely important discovery which proved to be the answer to the problem. After diluting the medicinal substance in water or alcohol, he vigorously shook the bottle containing the resulting dilution. He called this shaking *succussion*. The whole process of alternately diluting and shaking the medicinal substance he called *potentization* or *dynamization*. The resulting remedy was not only freed from toxicity, but to his amazement its curative powers were actually increased, as use in clinical practice proved.

The power in potentization

How could it be that a substance became *more* powerful the more it was diluted and succussed (or potentized), especially when the process of potentization was repeated beyond the time when any material portion of the substance remained? Hahnemann explained this by saying that during the process of potentization the material portion of the substance was decreased and the vital energy contained within was correspondingly increased or roused into activity. The vigorous process of potentization seemed to act as a catalyst, releasing the inner vital energy of the substance which had been concealed within the physical structure. Hahnemann found that his new system of medicine worked brilliantly in clinical practice and so returned to the practice of medicine, this time using homoeopathy.

In 1812 an epidemic of typhoid spread throughout Napoleon's army. Hahnemann treated 180 cases, of which only one died, and through this event homoeopathy spread through Europe.

It is likely that Hahnemann had come across the law of similars elsewhere in various guises as it had been mentioned by various scholars and physicians from the time of Hippocrates onwards.

Dilution and potentization of remedies

Hahnemann first considered that distilled water, alcohol and lactose (milk sugar) were medicinally inert, so he diluted the medicines in these media. If the remedy was soluble in water or alcohol he mixed one part of the substance with ninety-nine parts of the liquid and submitted the dilution to thirty vigorous succussions. In other words he banged the dilution on a leatherbound book thirty times. The resulting solution was called the first centesimal potency or 1c. He then mixed one drop of this solution with ninety-nine drops of the water or alcohol and submitted it to another thirty succussions, and called it the second centesimal potency or 2c. This he did up to thirty times to produce the 30c potency. This is called the centesimal scale. Today the whole process is usually carried out by machines and dilutions up to and beyond 100,000 are made.

The first six or more dilutions are usually carried out on the decimal scale. This means that one part of the drug is diluted in nine parts of the inert medium (water or alcohol). These dilutions are denominated by an *x* following the number, i.e. 1x, 2x, etc. For potencies beyond 6x the centesimal scale is usually used. Generally, the number alone on a remedy indicates the centesimal scale. For example, Acon 30 means the 30th potency carried out on the centesimal scale.

The implications of this discovery are staggering. Clearly this phenomenon cannot be explained by ordinary chemical analysis. These remedies are so diluted that not even one molecule of the original substance is left and yet the actual clinical results demonstrate beyond a doubt that an active influence remains – an influence which acts to cure a sick person quickly and permanently without side effects. Hahnemann found in clinical practice that even people suffering from deep-seated chronic dis-eases were beneficially affected by the correctly prescribed, potentized remedy.

An energy medicine

It must have become obvious to Hahnemann at this point that he had stumbled across an 'energy' medicine, as chemical analysis could detect no material substance whatsoever in his remedies. From this he deduced that the remedy, consisting solely of energy, could not be affecting the physical body directly. He considered that there must be an energizing principle to man which animated the physical body and which, if disturbed, caused disagreeable symptoms to be manifested. It was on this level that the potentized remedies had their initial effect We refer to this as the *dynamic level* and the energizing principle as the *vital force*.

Homoeopathy involves the ability to see life in all its forms as a whole connected picture; all physical phenomena being a reflection or result of the unmanifest which cannot be perceived with our limited physical sense organs, but can be seen to exist by its effects on the physical world.

Advanced thinkers throughout the ages have become more aware of the true nature of life and some of the laws governing it. This greater awareness has revealed methods of furthering potential and creating a more harmonious development within humanity. Through the use of this knowledge and awareness, methods of obtaining more abundant wholesome life have been developed.

Through this greater awareness Samuel Hahnemann observed that good health was not only reliant upon external influences such as hygiene and diet, but required a harmonious development within the individual.

The true nature of mankind

Homoeopathy recognizes the true nature of mankind to be that of a spiritual being. The body and mind, which is believed by the old school to be all there is to a person, is seen as a reflection of the inner man. All living things have both an outer, physical portion and an inner, vital portion which we cannot see, hear or feel, but which makes its presence known by its results in the physical world. The vital force occupies the same space as the physical body, animates and controls it and, given no opposition, will maintain the physical body in perfect health.

The vital force works ceaselessly for the highest good of the whole person, always trying to repel harmful influences and to absorb those things which give strength to the being, always adapting the being to changes and maintaining order and unity.

In a state of true health there is freedom and order, all parts working for the good of the whole. In this condition the vital force can repair and adapt the body without limit.

The real meaning of symptoms

A symptom is the outward sign of the inner dis-ease of the vital force, which is struggling to throw out those harmful forces or patterns of behaviour which threaten to harm the whole being.

The signs of acute dis-ease, which are usually eliminative processes, are the signs that the vital force is working actively

Extracts from the *Organon*

Hahnemann describes the properties of the vital force in aphorisms 9, 10 and 11 of his book, the *Organon:*

The healthy condition

Aphorism 9: In the healthy condition of man, the spiritual vital force, the dynamism that animates the material body, rules with unbounded sway and retains all the parts of the organism in admirable, harmonious, vital operation, as regards both sensations and functions, so that our indwelling, reason-gifted mind can freely employ this living, healthy instrument for the higher purposes of our existence.

The vital life principle

Aphorism 10: The material organism without the vital force is capable of no sensation, no function, no self-preservation; it derives all sensations and performs all the functions of life solely by means of the immaterial being (the vital principle) which animates the material organism in health and in dis-ease.

The dis-eased condition

Aphorism 11: When a person falls ill, it is only this spiritual, self-acting vital force, everywhere present in his organism, that is primarily deranged by the dynamic influence upon it of a morbific agent inimical to life; it is only the vital principle, deranged to such an abnormal state, that can furnish the organism with its disagreeable sensations and incline it to the irregular processes which we call dis-ease; for, as a power invisible in itself, and only recognizable by its effects on the organism, its morbid derangement only makes itself known by the manifestation of dis-ease in the sensations and functions of those parts of the organism exposed to the senses of the observer and physician, that is, by morbid symptoms, and in no other way can it make itself known.

Contained within these aphorisms are the answers to many questions concerning the nature of health and dis-ease. Please consider them carefully. Digest them thoroughly before continuing further. Try to understand what Hahnemann actually meant. His thinking was far beyond his time and even today is considered controversial. There is much to be learned from the study of these three aphorisms.

to restore order. If the process is not suppressed, and the vital force is strong enough to complete the process of elimination and renewal, then a greater degree of health follows. However, if the wrong kind of living habits are followed over a length of time the whole being is affected adversely in one way or another, resulting in a chronic state of dis-ease. This is an attempt by the vital force to maintain an equilibrium.

The laws discovered by Samuel Hahnemann

Homoeopathy aims to heal a person by strengthening and nourishing the weakened vital force so that it is able to free the individual from the morbific influence and restore order throughout the whole person. To restore a person to health homoeopathy follows the laws discovered by Samuel Hahnemann.

1. *Similia similibus curantur* (Like cures like). A substance which produces certain symptoms when given to a healthy person will, when given to a sick person who is producing very similar symptoms, remove those symptoms and restore the person to health.
2. *Potentization.* A process of repeatedly diluting and succussing a substance in an inert medium. This process was found to increase the power of the substance. As all living things have a vital force within, so the process of potentization seems to release the energy within the substance which then pervades the inert medium. As homoeopathy is aimed at the vital force within the individual, so the pure energy of the remedy, when given to a person to whom it is homoeopathic, will stimulate the weakened vital force at which it is aimed. Being of the same nature it is able to stimulate and nourish the vital force which is then able to perform its work properly and harmonize the whole person.

3. Homoeopathy – A Holistic Approach

The work of the homoeopathic prescriber

Homoeopathy is a holistic therapy which effects a cure by treating the whole person as an individual. The task of the prescriber is to discover the individuality of the patient assessed on the *totality* of the symptoms, with particular regard being paid to the characteristic, striking or unexpected symptoms. These individualize the patient's response to the harmful influence which has disturbed them in the first place. Using the law of similars, the curative remedy can then be found.

Using the law of similars

All potentized remedies have been 'proved' on healthy volunteers. These 'provings' provide us with the individualized symptom pictures of a great many remedies. For example Belladonna, when taken in small doses over a period of time by a prover, causes disturbances on all levels. Mentally, there would be anger, intensity and restlessness. Their senses would be extremely acute. In extreme cases the prover would be noisy, delirious and talk fast. Physically they would experience throbbing and pulsating pains. Symptoms would come on with great suddenness. There would be intense dry, burning heat with redness. Their oversensitivity would extend to light, noise and pressure. Also to touch, particularly to the head. It can cause a sore throat which is swollen, dry, burning hot and bright red. The fever would also be hot and dry and the skin would be burning to the touch. Perspiration would appear suddenly and disappear just as suddenly. This is a brief summary of a prover's report on taking Belladonna which clearly shows the individualized or characteristic symptoms of this remedy in a marked degree.

Using our knowledge of the law of similars we could use this remedy if an individual was experiencing similar symptoms on the mental, emotional and physical levels. For example the patient may be suffering from an extreme and violent headache which had come on with great suddenness, accompanied by great agitation on all levels. A fever may have broken out with great heat, dryness and a bright red colour to the skin. The orthodox diagnosis could be scarlet fever. To the homoeopath this diagnosis would be of little use, as another sufferer from scarlet fever may not have this general wildness, violence and agitation.

These characteristic symptoms help to individualize the case and point to Belladonna. Without these characteristic symptoms another remedy would be indicated, even though the orthodox diagnosis remains the same.

It would be of no use to isolate one part of the case, for example the headache, and prescribe on this symptom alone, as many other remedies can produce a violent, throbbing headache. If one were to prescribe in this way suppression could be the result. It is the *totality* of the symptoms which individualize the patient and therefore point towards the curative remedy. The name of the dis-ease from the homoeopathic standpoint is the name of the curative remedy.

Any medicine or therapy which removes symptoms from an isolated part without the patient experiencing a greater degree of general well-being is usually a palliative or suppressant. This sort of symptomatic prescribing can be necessary in certain circumstances, as for example when the problem is an injury. One would not seek to cure a broken leg with a potentized remedy – external treatment is necessary, although one would give a remedy also to stimulate the body's inherent healing abilities.

However, when the cause is within, the cure *must* proceed from within, otherwise, although a palliative or suppressant may eradicate the symptoms, the cause will remain. When a patient feels better in themselves, it is a sign that the cause has been removed and the cure is proceeding in the right direction, from the inside to the outside, and will then continue in an ordered way to heal the outermost external parts.

A holistic point of view

Homoeopathy is a holistic approach to health, based on the concept that man is an integrated whole, who in his natural state could be living on this earth in perfect harmony, both within himself and with the universe surrounding him. He could be living a natural, balanced, loving, creative life, complementing and aiding nature as nature is complementing and aiding him.

The holistic view perceives man as a whole being – body, mind and spirit. Those parts which cannot be perceived with the physical senses show their presence and their very nature by the effect they produce in the parts which can be perceived by the physical senses. In health the vital force maintains harmony and order throughout the organism under all circumstances, leading to a feeling of well-being and a creative and optimistic outlook. In sickness the vital force is disturbed and is unable to hold the organism in perfect equilibrium and so symptoms are produced.

From this holistic point of view, it is of no use to aim treatment solely at, say, a hand which is exhibiting an eruption and to apply a cream to the eruption in order to make it disappear. With that type of treatment the eruption may well disappear, but the patient will not be any better, the cause remains and if this is not also dealt with the eruption may appear again at a later date or may manifest itself in another way on a deeper level. When an eruption is caused to disappear by the use of an external application, one should ask oneself, 'Where did it go?', 'Is the cause removed?', 'Is the patient cured?'. The aim of homoeopathy, and indeed all truly holistic medicine, is to cure the patient, not just to get rid of the symptoms. Dis-ease symptoms will always disappear as a natural result of the laws of cause and effect when the *patient* is cured. The symptoms arose as a result of dis-ease, or dis-harmony, on an inner level of the patient and will just as naturally disappear as a result of ease and harmony having been re-established on that same inner level.

A consideration of susceptibility

A deranged or weakened vital force, or life energy, causes the individual to become susceptible to the various harmful influences which surround us all. Everyone is exposed to germs, bacteria, viruses, etc.; they reside within our bodies quite harmlessly, without any adverse symptoms being produced. It is only when a weakened or disturbed vital force produces susceptibility to these influences that they become harmful to us. Being unable to deal with them effectively, symptoms are produced. Or, in other words, a symptom *picture* is produced. In a 'flu epidemic one should not ask 'Why is it that so many people are affected?', when the more interesting question is 'Why is it that some people are not affected?'. An individual with a strong and ordered life energy will repel all harmful influences and will be the one who remains healthy and cheerful whilst all around succumb.

As the morbific influences do exist, and as they cannot be annihilated by force, as forceful means of annihilating germs and viruses only succeed in those germs and viruses becoming immune and evolving into generally stronger and more complex varieties, it would seem sensible to direct our efforts at strengthening the vital force of the individual, thereby removing susceptibility. You would no doubt agree that prevention is better than cure.

Benefits of the right remedy

Usually the first benefit noticed after the administration of the appropriate remedy is that the person feels better in themself and experiences a greater degree of well-being, even though the symptoms may remain for a short while. This is a sign that cure is proceeding in the right direction. The individual is better, their inner vitality is healed. Once the vital force is flowing harmoniously throughout their being, it stimulates the body's natural defence mechanism and a perfectly ordered chain reaction is begun which proceeds to effect the cure.

Dis-ease – lack of ease

Dis-ease is not only a physical pathological state. We write it with a hyphen and it is what it sounds like – a lack of ease – and it can exist on any level – spiritual, mental, emotional or physical. The creation of health means that a tendency towards and susceptibility, to pathological states is actually removed. Positive, vital force or life energy flows throughout the being and harmony and order prevail.

A new way of thinking

The study of homoeopathy involves a slight re-arranging of well-worn grooves of thinking. A moment's thought will help you realize that the words 'health' and 'dis-ease' are generally used without any thought as to their true meaning. Health is more than simply the absence of obvious symptoms. Health is freedom on all levels of the being. It is a positive state. The aim of homoeopathy is the creation of health.

4. Homoeopathic Philosophy

What is the vital force?

The energizing principle that homoeopaths call the vital force pervades all living things. J.T. Kent, master homoeopath of the nineteenth century, describes some of its qualities in his book *Lectures on Homoeopathic Philosophy*:

1. It is endowed with formative intelligence, i.e. it intelligently operates and forms the economy of the human organism.
2. It is constructive, it keeps the body continually constructed and reconstructed, but when the opposite is true, when the vital force from any cause withdraws from the body, we see that the forces that are in the body being turned loose, are destructive.
3. It is subject to changes, in other words it may be flowing in order or disorder, it may be sick or normal.
4. It dominates and controls the body it occupies.
5. It has adaption. That the individual has an adaption to his environment is not questioned – but what is it that adapts itself to the environment? The dead body cannot. When we reason, we see that the vital force adapts itself to its surrounds and thus the human body is kept in a state of order in the cold or in the heat, in the wet and damp and under all circumstances.

Experiencing the vital force

As the vital force is dynamic in nature we can only know of it by the results it produces on the mental, emotional and physical levels. Subjectively we can experience the vital force working within us by our fluctuations in energy and sense of general well-being. We can know of its condition by our ability to adapt to changes. If this is poor the vital force is not flowing freely and the results of this obstruction are shown in the symptoms produced in varying degrees on all or any of the levels mentioned previously.

The vital force is that which reacts firstly to any harmful stimulus of whatever nature. It is only then that any or all of the other levels are affected. This will, of course, depend on the ability of the vital force to adapt the organism to the influences surrounding it (see Figure 1). Knowing this, it would seem prudent to direct our therapeutic measures at the vital force and not at any of the correspondingly affected levels which have exhibited symptoms.

As the nature of the vital force is dynamic, it would follow that the nature of the remedies should be of this 'simple substance', as it is referred to by J.T. Kent. In homoeopathy we have such remedies and, through the observations of Samuel Hahnemann, the understanding to use them efficaciously when they are called for by the language of symptoms.

The vital force's mode of action

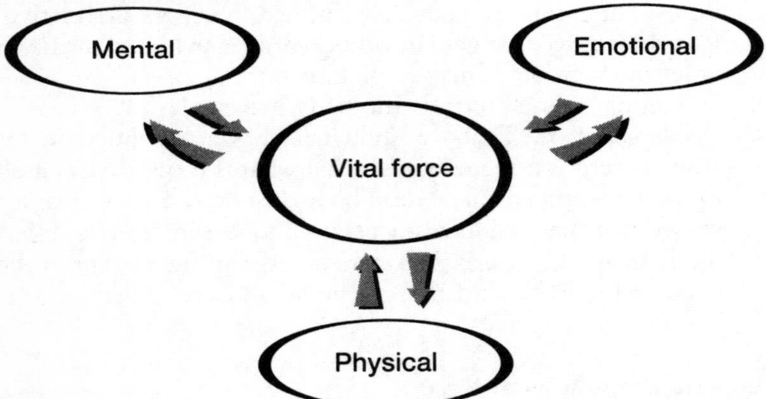

Figure 1

Figure 1 demonstrates the relationship of the vital force to the organism as a whole. Notice how the vital aspects of the organism can only affect each other through the mediation of the vital force. The vital force is the balancing, harmonizing and activating centre of the individual and it is here that any attempt at encouraging energy and health should be aimed. It is of course acceptable to help each individual aspect of the being with the appropriate means as long as the vital force is aided in its activities and not hindered. This is where the holistic view is essential.

If the vital force encounters a harmful influence to which it is susceptible, then the individual's defence mechanism will activate, producing symptoms. The defence mechanism would then attempt to bring the vital force back to its threshold. The question of the vital force's threshold is discussed a little later on in the text. If the vital force is strong (see Figure 3) we would repel the harmful influence without any apparent disruption; that is, we would adapt to the change. In other words, we would not be susceptible to the influence.

Energy, health and dis-ease

The dynamic or energy question is an elusive one as it is not directly observable. However, the results it produces on the material plane raise many questions. How can something without substance affect substance? These considerations point us towards the ideas of energy, vibration and resonance for the answer.

There have been numerous attempts at explaining energy, but few have achieved this successfully because energy in its pure form exists on a different plane of reality from the material one that we all know so well. We shall refer to this level as the *dynamic plane*. We have ample proof of its existence by the results it has on the material level of life but to prove this scientifically can be a difficult job. As yet, man has not been able to create an instrument capable of perceiving its totality. It can be measured, but again only by a reflex action – that is, by its effects.

Consider gravity, for instance. We know it exists by the fact that we have weight and don't fly off the planet into space. We can measure its force by the means of sophisticated instruments, but we still cannot show the force of gravity as existing by studying the force directly, because we cannot see, smell or hear it. Magnetism is another example of this.

Man today can be his own worst enemy. He can accept such

things as gravity and magnetism without a second thought, as they cannot be denied. However, energy medicine and therapies which utilize the forces around and within us are met with great scepticism and, in some instances, ridicule. Why is this when the results are as clear as the other examples mentioned?

Energy is necessary for life. It is the foundation of life. Without it all would collapse. It is prior to everything but is not separate. The material/physical part of life is dependent on the energy which pervades it for its shape or form. Take away the energy and the form collapses or is subjected to the natural forces of decay. This can occur in varying degrees of intensity. If the energy source is weak we get a signal on the material level and an alarm will sound in the language of symptoms. (See Figure 2.)

It would seem more advantageous to prevent rather than to have to cure. The question is, why is it that we are susceptible to imbalance on the energy level in the first place, and how does this imbalance occur?

Things are not all they appear to be

It is known that nothing is as solid as it may appear. Everything is made up of a multitude of atoms moving at incredible speed. This movement creates vibrations which are generally imperceptible. These vibrations vary in frequency within the living organism, affected by other vibrations which may be caused by a physical or dynamic experience.

For example, an emotional shock – dynamic influence – sets up waves which influence the vital force. This in turn may affect the mental, emotional or physical levels according to the strength of the shock and the degree of resistance (see Figure 2).

We are all individuals; no one is supposed to be like anyone else. This can help us to understand why everyone has their own individual level of health. There is a certain area where the degrees of health are difficult to distinguish, but nevertheless, no one is on exactly the same level as anyone else. We have indicated that everything is made up of a multitude of atoms, all moving at incredible speed. That movement, or vibration, has an optimum frequency. That is, all things have a certain rate of vibration at which stability is assumed. This optimum frequency maintains a certain physical form. The atoms are held in a certain pattern which create the physical form that we see. If the vibrational frequency were to change, the physical form must change also as its pattern of existence is altered.

Any harmful influence – whether it be a virus or shock or whatever – could resonate with any level of the vital force, depending on the degree of similarity of their vibrational frequencies (see Figure 3). The degree of reaction to the morbific influence depends on its intensity and the degree of health at the time.

If the vibration of the harmful influence closely matched that of level C and the vital force was at level A the effect would be mild, if felt at all. If the harmful influence and the level of the vital force were similar, a resonance would be created and could push the vital force beyond its threshold, causing symptoms to be produced.

The health threshold

The vital force has a certain range of vibrations within which it can move without noticeable symptoms being produced. If it were to move beyond this range the defence mechanism would activate, producing symptoms. For ease of explanation we will consider the extreme ends of the range to be plus and minus. When we are closer to the plus end of the range the subjective experience will be one of extreme vitality and well-being. When we are closer to the minus end we will experience less vitality and feel 'a few degrees under'. When the vital force is closer to this minus end we are more susceptible to the millions of harmful influences which surround us.

We have discussed how all things vibrate at their own frequency and vibrational frequencies can affect one another. So, bearing this in mind, it does not seem improbable that we ourselves can also be affected by vibrational influences. The following diagram may be of help in understanding this further.

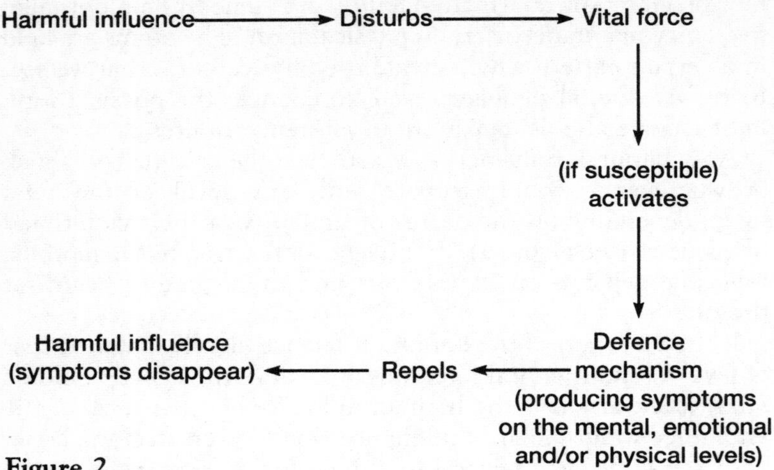

Figure 2

Figure 2 illustrates the sequence of events which occur when the vital force is disturbed by a harmful influence to which it is susceptible. (If it is not susceptible no reaction is experienced.) Symptoms are produced as the defence mechanism is activated, as it works to repel or inhibit the effect of the harmful influence. If it is successful in its task the frequency of the vital force returns to within its threshold and the symptoms disappear. If it is not totally successful an equilibrium is maintained and some symptoms remain.

Orthodox medical treatment aims to eradicate the symptoms without recognizing the dynamic disturbance. This kind of symptomatic prescribing can change symptoms or add new symptoms as the defence mechanism reacts to the new disturbance (often termed drug side effects). If cure occurs under these circumstances it is due to an accidental resonance, or the individual's vital force has sufficient vitality to return to within its threshold despite the interference.

Dis-ease considered from a vibrational viewpoint

An external vibrational frequency, with the physical form of a germ or a non-physical form such as shock or grief, resonates or interacts with the individual's vibrational frequency, if it is susceptible to it. This harmful influence disturbs the equilibrium and forces the individual's vital force vibration over its threshold. The organism, in its attempt to survive, produces symptoms in order to arrest the deterioration. These symptoms are seen by the holistic practitioner as cries for help from the organism's intelligent life energy.

The physical form of a glass can be changed dramatically by a certain vibrational frequency in the form of sound. In fact the glass's optimum frequency will be so altered by the stimulus of another frequency that it can no longer hold its physical form and is shattered. It could be said that it has been forced beyond its threshold. It only has a certain frequency range within which it can maintain its form.

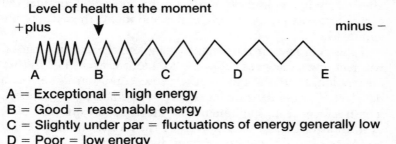

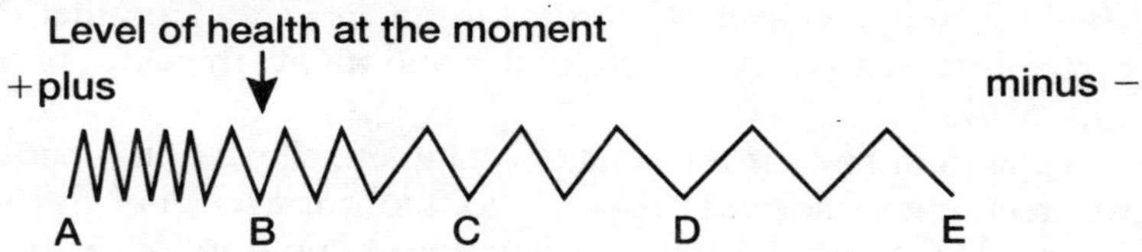

A = Exceptional = high energy
B = Good = reasonable energy
C = Slightly under par = fluctuations of energy generally low
D = Poor = low energy
E = Very poor = very low energy

Figure 3

If you push the vital force outside its threshold it cannot return before it has reached its eliminative climax; this could be considered as a throwing off of the harmful influence. This is usually observed as a fever reaching its height, vomiting or diarrhoea or any other strong, successful, eliminative effort on the mental, emotional and/or physical level. It then follows that the individual recovers if, unlike the glass, they have not been destroyed in the process. If the vital force is not strong enough there is no eliminative climax and therefore it does not return to within its threshold. Instead we see the development of a chronic situation or what may be termed twilight health. If the vital force is too weak to complete the process by itself it can be helped by a similar vibrational frequency in the form of the homoeopathic similimum – this will create a controlled climaxing of symptoms. Following this the vital force would return to within its threshold, i.e. there would be a return to health.

The homoeopathic similimum would give sufficient strength to the vital force, enabling it to naturally complete its process of elimination in an intelligent manner, i.e. without the danger of the organism shattering like the glass. We believe that this is why homoeopathic remedies create an aggravation, if selected correctly. The vital force, once freed from its struggle, is then able to return to within its threshold, often moving several notches up the scale of health towards the plus end. This is why, after an acute condition which has culminated in a successful elimination, one feels far better than before it occurred. It is, in a sense, a rebound action. It is a natural law that anything, after reaching its pinnacle, returns to its opposite. Consider the cycle of the seasons, the cycle of day and night, the cycle of life and death.

If the vital force is too weak to complete the action a person will feel several degrees below par for months even though they are no longer in the grip of the acute condition. There is a deadlock. A suitable stimulus is needed to change the situation. The homoeopathic similimum does much good work here also, even though it could have prevented the months of malaise if it had been given at the first signs of disharmony.

Be aware

Please do not attempt to treat people suffering from chronic conditions as more information than this book can supply is required.

5. The Course of Dis-ease and the Return to Health

The move to harmony

The vital force, when strong and healthy, does its proper work, and will maintain a state of harmony throughout the being, ensuring that all functions are efficiently carried out: digestion, assimilation and elimination will go on perfectly; all parts will be kept nourished and clean; injuries will be sent the necessary materials for repair; and all the separate parts will be caused to function together in harmony, for the highest good of the whole being. The whole being will be kept in a state of health, freedom, vitality and ease; and can therefore freely express the higher qualities of life, such as love, truth, creativity, etc.

If the vital force is strong and is flowing energetically and harmoniously through the organism, then the being will manifest all the signs of optimum health. Each person has their own totally individual nature, each has his or her own strengths and weaknesses. Harmful habits may be in the mental sphere – as in negative thoughts and beliefs; in the emotional sphere – as in negative emotions; and in the physical sphere – as in harmful physical habits, such as overeating, eating of devitalized foods, excessive indulgence in stimulants and tranquillizers of various kinds, lack of fresh air and exercise, etc. All of these things can weaken the vital force and obstruct its free flow. A state of disorder is the result. The body is then readily susceptible to any harmful influence to which it is exposed. There is under or oversecretion; assimilation, digestion and elimination are not carried out properly; toxic wastes pile up in the weakest parts of the organism.

The cleansing process in chronic dis-ease

At this stage, when the vital force finds the burden too much to bear, if it has the necessary energy or is in some way stimulated, then it energetically sets to work to restore order, so that it may once more flow throughout the organism unobstructed. The result of this restoration to order is a cleansing process, involving a lot of dust and disturbance. The vital force mobilizes the defence mechanism of the organism, which sweeps through the system, firstly cleansing and putting into order the parts most necessary for life. The individual could experience mental, emotional and physical disruption. This could result in emotional outbursts, intellectual reasoning and organ cleansing. Due to this cleansing process debris is swept into the bloodstream and temporarily adversely affects less important parts of the organism. This process can take various forms such as colds, fevers, diarrhoea, skin eruptions, headaches, etc., but they are all varieties of the same action. As toxins are swept from within to without to be eliminated, they may give rise to a wide variety of symptoms of an acute nature. A state of twilight health is being exchanged for a state of acute dis-ease. The vital force, in its efforts to restore order and gain a notch up the scale towards optimum health, causes these symptoms to appear by activating the defence mechanism. They can be seen as the external sign of the inner dis-ease of the vital force adapting to change.

If the vital force is not aided in its eliminative efforts, and particularly if the defence mechanism is forcibly suppressed (which can be done in many ways), then the result will eventually be a state of chronic dis-ease. The vital force will maintain a kind of equilibrium within the being and the symptoms produced will be the only way it can maintain this equilibrium.

A weakened vital force needs stimulation

In the case of chronic dis-ease the vital force needs to be stimulated into activity. It has become too weakened and disturbed to correct the situation without aid. The correct homoeopathic remedy does much good work here, as do controlled fasting and eliminative diets. The road along which the individual has travelled to reach this state of chronic dis-ease must be retraced. Homoeopathic treatment, combined with nutritional awareness, will stimulate the vital force, which will instigate the return to order. It will sometimes involve a re-emerging of old, suppressed symptoms, although this is not always easily seen as the form they take is not always the same as at the time when they were suppressed. During this process the symptoms which are re-experienced will last a much shorter time than they did originally, usually a matter of a few hours or days. The power of the correct homoeopathic remedy to restore order to the person is great. The remedy itself is dynamic and acts as a catalyst to the vital force, instigating it to act. Understanding usually comes after the administration of the correct homoeopathic remedy and the individual then begins to aid rather than hinder the vital force in its wonderful work.

Herings Law of Cure

The direction of cure is from within out, from above down, from a more important organ to a less important organ, in reverse order as the symptoms have appeared.

The natural healing process

In many acute cases the individual's vital force has sufficient vitality to return to within its threshold after a short time – aided only by rest and abstinence from certain foods. If the individual listens to their own inner intelligence and obeys the instinctive measures that the vital force prescribes, all can be well within a few days. Are we not all aware of the desire for rest and the aversion to certain foods when we are feeling 'low'?

This natural healing process occurs more readily in individuals who are in tune with their inner selves; those in whom the inner wise voice of the vital force has not been consistently ignored or too weakened by suppression. Perhaps you can understand how this happens when you think that consistently being too busy to

Figure 4

Homoeopathic treatment stimulates and increases the energy of the vital force which in turn motivates the organism to eliminate toxins, repair damage and generally remove the obstructions to a higher level of health. At this point the individual may experience a health crisis.

This rational process goes through particular stages based on the organism's inherent understanding of that which is best for its survival and evolvement. A 'health crisis' always give rise to an intensifying of symptoms on the mental, emotional and/or physical levels (not always so apparent in acute cases as the symptoms are already at a high pitch).

The correct homoeopathic remedy will bring the individual safely through such a crisis resulting in a higher level of health and a lowering of susceptibility to dis-ease.

Suppression may be brought about through negative mental attitudes, emotional obstruction, unholistic therapies, drugs, poor nutritional considerations, in fact anything which prevents elimination and free flow. The result would be a build-up of toxins within the organism which would obstruct the action of the vital force. Eventually more energy would be required than was available to clear the toxins and maintain the organism in a state of equilibrium. This would result in a 'health crisis'. Suppressive action at this point would lower the level of health even more, increasing the individual's susceptibility to more serious dis-ease.

obey the organism's call to pass a bowel motion results in no daily call being given – hence constipation.

Early warning signs

We all know the type of person who is always too busy to rest or to eat properly when all the signs are indicating that they need to do this. Very often they are forced by extreme measures, instigated by the obstructed vital force, to do as they are told.

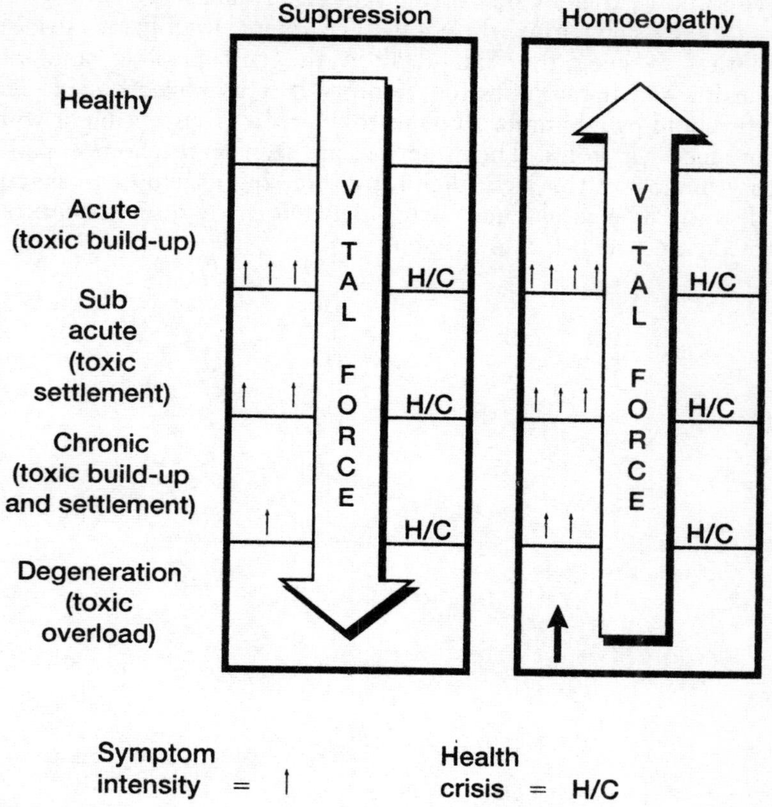

Figure 4

For example, the overworked, undernourished person forced to bed-rest due to susceptibility to some infection; the prolapsed disc that was but a little (ignored) twinge, not many months before; or the indigestion that precedes the ulcer.

Homoeopathy can not only prevent these extremes becoming a reality but, being dynamic in nature, can give strength to the vital force, which in turn will accomplish the move back to within its threshold in a remarkably short time. The timely administration of the homoeopathic similimum can shorten the course of acute conditions, thereby preventing prolonged suffering.

So, to summarize, the vital force, being intelligent, strives always to keep the individual in the best possible state of health and harmonious functioning. If it is moved outside its threshold by a harmful stimulus to which it is susceptible it will produce symptoms. The symptoms are seen by the homoeopath as attempts of the vital force to restore equilibrium or to signal distress. The vital force, being dynamic in nature, requires a medicine which is also dynamic.

Part Two

Please read Part Two VERY CAREFULLY, *two or three times at least, before using your remedies.*

6. The Work of the Homoeopathic Prescriber

Taking the case

In order to prescribe a homoeopathic remedy in any given situation you must first 'take the case'. This will enable you to discover the individuality of the patient, or the individual way in which they are expressing their dis-ease. Anything that is a change from the patient's normal healthy state can be a sign or symptom. The aim is to discover anything you can about the patient and the way that they are expressing their symptoms through observation and questioning. Listen carefully to your patient's story. The information you gather may relate to their physical condition, their general condition, and/or their mental/emotional condition. Also consider contributory, aggravating and ameliorating factors such as a cold wind, a soaking, bad meat, a disappointment, movement, touch, noise, etc. The totality of all these symptoms is called the *symptom picture* and it individualizes the patient's suffering.

Individualizing the patient

We are generally used to looking at someone suffering from disagreeable symptoms with a view to putting a name to their condition. This limits our possibilities of seeing the patient's individuality. The symptoms which enable us to name a condition are common to the 'disease' or orthodox diagnosis, but do not help us to find the correct remedy homoeopathically. For example, fever, sore throat, aching limbs, chills and lack of appetite are symptoms common to the condition diagnosed as influenza. From a homoeopathic viewpoint, however, several people all suffering from influenza may each need a different remedy, according to how they are expressing their symptom picture, or, in other words, their individuality.

Common and characteristic symptoms

A homoeopathic prescriber needs to expand their view to incorporate into the picture any sign or symptom or other relevant factor which is *individual to the patient*. The symptoms which express the individuality of the patient are called *characteristic symptoms*, and it is these which are most useful for finding the appropriate remedy. One patient with the common symptoms of influenza may be individualized from another by their characteristic symptoms. One may be anxious and fearful whereas another may be lethargic and drowsy. One may be worse for any movement while another is restless. One may look pink and dusky while another looks bright red. One may be thirstless while another cannot get enough to drink. These types of symptoms individualize one patient from another and are characteristic of certain remedies.

Remember there is no such thing as a homoeopathic remedy for influenza. A remedy only becomes homoeopathic when given to a patient whose symptom picture it matches or is most similar to.

As we have said, if you take just the patient's common symptoms, such as headache, sore throat, stomach ache, etc., you would have a choice of many remedies and no way of knowing which one to choose, as many remedies cover these common symptoms. The more you individualize, by using the characteristic symptoms of the patient, the more you narrow down your choice of remedies. Through observation and questions you will be able to determine the patient's symptom picture. The best way to learn what to look for is to study the symptom pictures of the remedies. As you become familiar with the *remedy pictures* in this book you will soon be able to recognize which remedy picture your patient's symptom picture reminds you of. You will see, for example, that Bryonia is characteristically much worse from the slightest movement and is extremely thirsty for long cold drinks.

Apis mel. has burning, stinging pains and is generally worse from heat of any kind. By studying the remedies you will see what there is in the remedy pictures which can be matched with the symptom picture of the patient. Generally speaking the remedy chosen should have most of the characteristic symptoms of the patient, although the patient will *never have all of the symptoms of the remedy.* Study of other books, such as those in the Further Reading list at the back of this book, will enable those of you who wish to take these studies further, to expand on your knowledge of remedies.

Observations and questions

Much information can be gathered from observation alone. One can tell a lot from the appearance of the patient – pale or flushed, sweaty or dry, hot or chilly, bright red, rosy or dusky pink, one cheek brilliant red and hot, the other pale and cool, and so on. Then there is the expression – fearful, anxious, confused, irritable, depressed, dull, drowsy, heavy, indifferent, angry, etc. The mental and emotional state is particularly important if it is different from when the patient is well. It may be revealed by their appearance, the sound of their voice, the things they say and the way they say them, by their actions, by their activity or lack of activity – still, mild, listless, restless, excitable, tossing and turning anxiously, making a lot of noise, or indifferent, wanting nothing except to be left alone and becoming touchy when disturbed, wanting company, fuss and attention, or becoming angry and embarrassed from fuss and attention.

Note if there are any times of day that they are worse, or sides of the body that are particularly affected. Also, any particular odours – of sweat, breath, feet, etc – should be taken into account. Note if there is sweat only on particular places – only on the head, only on the feet, only on uncovered parts, etc. If they are hot, what kind of heat is it? Dry, moist, burning, etc. What is the weather like? Has it had any effect on the patient?

Note the cause if it is known and pronounced – is it due to exposure to extremes of temperature; weather conditions of any sort – bitter cold, dry weather, warm damp weather, extreme heat, chilly weather after warm weather, etc? The cause may be due to many other things; shock, anger, nervous anticipation of a forthcoming event, a disappointment, over-excitement, lack of sleep, strains – whether mental or physical – prolonged exertion of a mental or physical nature, irritability, anger, frustration, embarrassment, and so on.

It is also usually necessary to ask questions in order to obtain as complete a symptom picture as possible. In some cases you will find a particularly characteristic symptom which points you directly towards the most suitable remedy. For example, extreme fright is characteristic of Aconite; complaints coming on after getting chilled when hot are characteristic of Dulcamara; pain which is worse on first movement and better for continued movement is characteristic of Rhus tox. Knowing the characteristic symptoms of the remedies will save you a lot of time when dealing with an actual situation. However, you should still make sure that the chosen remedy is similar to the whole symptom picture expressed by the patient.

Symptoms – order of importance

As we have said common symptoms are of least importance in helping you to decide on the remedy as they can be found in most cases and so do not help in the process of remedy selection. However, common symptoms can become more important if they are accompanied by a modifying factor. For example, a sore throat is a common symptom and therefore not very useful. However, a sore throat which is better from swallowing hard toast becomes a useful, guiding symptom. Similarly, a sore throat which is only on the right side gains in importance. Particular symptoms which are striking or unusual can be of more use in finding the remedy than common General or Mental/Emotional symptoms. However, as a general rule the order of importance of symptoms is as follows:

1. *Mental and emotional symptoms:* e.g. irritable, weepy, mild, irresolute, anxious, fearful, anticipatory, restless, etc.
2. *General symptoms:* these relate to the whole person and usually start with the prefix 'I', e.g. 'I feel chilly', 'I feel thirsty', 'I feel better in cool air'. Desires and aversions belong in this category.

3. *Particular symptoms:* these relate to specific parts and are usually prefixed with 'my', e.g. 'my hand is sore', 'my mouth is dry', 'my head aches'.
4. *Modalities*: these are circumstances or factors which modify the symptoms or the patient. You can ask what makes your patient feel better and what they do to obtain any relief from each of their symptoms, and also what aggravates each of their symptoms and makes them feel worse. Modalities are extremely useful for individualizing your patient and finding their remedy. They can turn a relatively unimportant and common symptom into a more important one. They can be applied to each symptom as well as to the patient as a whole, e.g. headache better from cool air (particular common symptom with a modality) and patient better from cool air (general modality).

The symptoms in your case which have a modality or are striking, unusual or unexpected can often lead you directly to a small selection of well-indicated remedies. A few examples of these types of symptoms are: burning pains better from heat (Arsenicum album); irritability – aggravated by consolation (Ignatia); sore throat better from swallowing rough foods (Ignatia); dry mouth without thirst (Pulsatilla, Gelsemium). These symptoms are very useful as they help to individualize the patient. It is often the factors which aggravate or ameliorate your patient or your patient's symptoms which can help you narrow down your remedy choice.

How to proceed

When observing or enquiring about the patient's symptoms, find out about the following.

Location: what is its exact position? Head, neck, stomach, fingers, etc.

Sensation: what does it feel like? Hot, numb, throbbing, stinging, etc.

Modalities: what makes the patient feel better or worse and what do they do to obtain any relief from each of the symptoms.

Cause: take note of the cause if it is obvious and definite as this can also point you towards the most likely remedy. For example a person who comes down with symptoms shortly after exposure to a bitterly cold wind may well require a dose of Aconite; a person who comes down with symptoms shortly after eating some spoiled meat may require Arsenicum album; a person obviously suffering from the effects of nervous anticipation may find they are helped by a dose of Gelsemium. These are all characteristics of these remedies. Reading your remedy pictures will help you to understand this more fully.

Use the remedies wisely

Please understand that the indications given in this guide are intended for use in the everyday common conditions that arise in any home from time to time. It is in no way intended to take the place of your experienced physician. If the situation is more serious, or symptoms persist, you must contact your doctor. This is not to say that one cannot administer an appropriate remedy whilst waiting for help to arrive.

Homoeopathic medicines do not interfere in any way with orthodox medicines, which may be knowingly or unknowingly, administered to the patient at the same time. However, the orthodox medicine may antidote the homoeopathic remedy.

7. Test Case Examples Using the Grid

Three test cases have been provided for you to try your skill. They are good practice cases and will help you to understand the practical aspects of case taking and finding the remedy. The answers to the cases can be found on page 110. The following completed example test case will give you the idea. To speed up case-taking, worse can be indicated by the sign < and better can be indicated by the sign > i.e. headache > cool air, headache < movement.

Case taking example

A man comes home from work, **complaining** of a **throbbing headache.** He complains constantly, all the while **restlessly** pacing the floor. He tells his wife that he **cannot stand the pain,** and in a **demanding** way, asks that she do something for him.

She enquires as to what may have brought on the headache. He replies in an **irritable manner**, that he was all right until he had this argument at work. He had become **angry** with the way his manager had treated him. It was after this that the headache came on. He also mentioned that after he had a **cup of coffee the headache seemed to get much worse.** When she asks where the pain is he tells her it is all over but **worse on one side** of his head.

He then starts to complain of being **hot and thirsty.** She asks what he would like to drink and he asks for tea, which he complains about when given. After one sip of the tea he pours it away and then uses the **warm cup to press against his head.** It helps the pain, he tells his astonished wife.

He then asks for a glass of water as he is still **very thirsty.** His wife considers him to be **capricious,** not knowing what he really wants. She tries to comfort him and feels that he is **clammy and hot.** When he is asked what the pain is like the husband says that he **can not stand it,** that it is excruciating, and demands she give him something to take the pain away. She decides to give him a remedy. What would she give him?

Here is a man with a head pain which he finds intolerable. He is extremely irate with it. The irritability is a very pronounced symptom and the wife must try to be objective otherwise she would react to this and probably would not see it as such. It is observed that the man's mental state is one of irritability, intolerance, capriciousness, over-sensitivity to pain, restlessness and impatience. He is certainly demanding. He had said that the head symptoms had come on suddenly after he had become angry with a work colleague. It was observed that warmth seemed to ameliorate the head pain. It was discovered that the pain was throbbing, one-sided and worse from coffee. He had made it known that he was hot and thirsty. It was discovered that the heat was of a clammy nature and that his thirst was mainly for water.

Now you make a list of all the presenting symptoms and then arrange them in order, considering all the modalities at the end. Note down the mode of onset and possible cause if known. To help you we have set it out below.

Mode of onset:	Sudden
Possible cause:	Anger
Mental/Emotional symptoms:	Restless, irritable, capricious, over-sensitive (to pain), demanding, impatient
General symptoms:	('I feel . . .') Hot and clammy, thirsty
Particular symptoms:	Headache – throbbing, one-sided
Modalities	
Mental/emotional:	< anger (poss cause)
Generals:	None
Particulars:	Headache < coffee, > warmth

Symptom Analysis Grid – Example A

	REMEDIES																				
SYMPTOMS	ACONITE	APIS MEL.	ARSENICUM ALB.	BELLADONNA	BRYONIA	CALCAREA CARB.	CARBO VEG.	CHAMOMILLA	CINA	DULCAMARA	GELSEMIUM	HEPAR SULPH.	IGNATIA	LYCOPODIUM	NUX VOM.	PULSATILLA	RHUS TOX.	SPONGIA	SULPHUR		
1. Sudden onset	√			√				√							√						
2. Possible cause-anger	√				√			√							√						
3. Restlessness	√	√	√	√				√						√	√		√		√		
4. Irritability	√	√	√	√	√	√		√	√	√		√		√	√	√	√		√		
5. Capricious					√			√	√	√									√		
6. Over-sensitive	√			√				√	√			√	√	√	√	√			√		
7. Demanding								√	√						√						
8. Impatient	√		√	√	√	√		√		√					√				√		
9. Hot and clammy								√													
10. Thirsty	√		√	√	√	√		√						√		√			√		
11. Headache – throbbing				√	√			√						√							
12. Headache – one sided								√													
13. Headache < coffee								√					√		√						
14. Headache > warmth								√							√						
15.																					
16.																					
17.																					
18.																					
19.																					
20.																					
SCORE	7	2	4	7	5	3	0	14	4	3	0	2	2	5	9	3	2	0	6		

This case is an obvious Chamomilla picture. With experience you will not need to list all the remedies. To help you learn the characteristics of the remedies included in this book, it is a good idea to include them all until you have gained sufficient experience to know which ones to leave out. You may also wish to include remedies in the grid which you have learnt from other sources.

Symptom analysis grid

To assist you in finding the remedy in any given case we have devised a symptom analysis grid. (See example A.)

You will probably not need to use this when you have become familiar with twenty or thirty remedy pictures, however it will help at the beginning.

Finding the Remedy Using the Grid

(a) List all the symptoms available in the left-hand column provided on your grid.

(b) Search through the remedy pictures in Part 3 of the book for any of the symptoms that have been listed. For example, starting with the first remedy, **Aconite**, we find it has the symptoms: **sudden onset, ailments from anger, restlessness, irritability, over-sensitive, impatient, thirsty**. (Note: **Aconite** is 'hot' but it is a dry heat, not the clammy warmth we have in our case example.)

(c) In the **Aconite column** make a tick in the boxes alongside each of the number listed symptoms i.e. **(1)** Sudden onset, **(2)** Possible cause – anger, **(3)** restlessness **(4)** irritability **(6)** over-sensitivity **(8)** impatience **(10)** thirsty. We have seven symptoms for Aconite so we write **'7' in the score column.**

(d) Turn back to Part 3 for further reference. Looking through the next remedy, **Apis mel.,** we find the symptoms: **(3)** restlessness **(4)** irritability. Make ticks in the two relevant boxes and write **'2' in the score** column. (Note: **Apis mel.** has head pains, but these are worse from heat, not better as is the case with our man.)

(e) Turn back to part 3 to read through the next remedy, **Arsenicum album.** Here we find the following symptoms: **(3)** restlessness, **(4)** irritable, **(8)** impatience, **(10)** thirsty. Make ticks in the relevant boxes in the Arsenicum column. Add up and enter the score in the score column. (Note: **Arsenicum alb.**

is better from warmth generally, however the **Arsenicum alb.** headache is usually better from cold water and cool air.)

(f) Continue this process with each remedy in turn, checking for symptoms, entering them into the grid by ticking the relevant numbered boxes in the relevant columns, and giving them a score by adding up each separate column. When you have completed the symptom analysis using the grid, you will find that several remedies have one or two of the symptoms, some have several, whilst the most similar remedy to the case example will have the most.

Selecting the remedy

The symptom analysis grid method has helped you to narrow down the choice of remedies by eliminating those which do not cover many of the symptoms. In our case example Chamomilla is the highest scoring of all the remedies used. Nux. vom. comes close behind. Always read through the highest scoring remedies carefully in order to select the remedy which is most similar to the patient you are treating.

If you find that two remedies seem to score equally and you cannot decide between them it may be that you have not obtained sufficient modalities or characteristic symptoms. In this case you will have to ask more searching questions. For example if they are both hot what type of heat is it? Aconite may be dry and hot whereas Chamomilla may be clammy and hot. Or if they both have a headache, what do they do to relieve it? Pulsatilla would be better from slow movement in the the cool air while Bryonia would be worse from any movement at all. If they are thirsty is it for sips like Arsenicum alb. or for long draughts like Bryonia?

The final choice is always made in terms of the remedy picture and its similarity as a whole to the patient's symptom picture, bearing in mind the question 'Is this patient suffering as if proving Chamomilla?' or whatever remedy you are considering.

Remember the grid is only a tool, which should be used to guide not to decide. Try and get a feel for the remedies, as each has

Symptom Analysis Grid

	REMEDIES																				
SYMPTOMS	ACONITE	APIS MEL.	ARSENICUM ALB.	BELLADONNA	BRYONIA	CALCAREA CARB.	CARBO VEG.	CHAMOMILLA	CINA	DULCAMARA	GELSEMIUM	HEPAR SULPH.	IGNATIA	LYCOPODIUM	NUX VOM.	PULSATILLA	RHUS TOX.	SPONGIA	SULPHUR		
1.																					
2.																					
3.																					
4.																					
5.																					
6.																					
7.																					
8.																					
9.																					
10.																					
11.																					
12.																					
13.																					
14.																					
15.																					
16.																					
17.																					
18.																					
19.																					
20.																					
SCORE																					

The reader has permission to photocopy this grid.

its own peculiarities, which you will come to recognize in your patients' expressions of their dis-ease.

Getting to know the remedies

You will soon find that the Aconite fear with panic and restlessness will strike you even before you have completed a list of symptoms and you will be led straight to the remedy by these *characteristics*. This will happen with the striking or unusual symptoms of other remedies also. You will be led to Gelsemium by seeing its image in a patient's dull, heavy, drowsy droopiness. You will also be led to Gelsemium when seeing nervous anticipation with trembling, relaxation and diarrhoea in a patient. You will be led to Belladonna by seeing its image in a patient, whether it be the dry, burning heat and redness which guides you to it or the characteristic anger and intensity. The clingy, tearful patient who wants your company all the time and requests cool air will lead you to the remedy Pulsatilla. In time you will begin to see that the remedies are like people, each having their own characteristics and individual ways of expressing themselves.

Finding the remedy – case examples

We have set three test cases for you to practise finding the remedy using the symptom analysis grids provided. Answers can be found on page 110.

The following case examples show the stages of working in order to find the remedy and give a good idea of how to arrive at the most suitable remedy. Firstly the case is given as it actually occurs; next, to make the case clearer, the presenting symptoms are arranged into a concise list with their mode of onset, possible cause, mentals and emotionals, generals, particulars and modalities. This gives us a clear symptom picture which we can compare with our remedy pictures in order to find the most similar.

It may help you to underline any symptoms which strike you as unusual or characteristic as they may well indicate one or two remedies to look up first. For example, in case example 1, under mentals, we find *fearful, restless* and *anxious*. None of these is particularly unusual. However, under generals we find *sudden onset*, which immediately eliminates remedies having a gradual onset and brings to mind a few remedies which are notable for *sudden onset*. Again under generals we find *came on after exposure to cold, dry wind*. This symptom also is characteristic of a few remedies and brings to mind those which are worth checking out first.

As you look through your remedy pictures, check out those remedies which have both *sudden onset* and *came on after exposure to cold, dry wind*. Whilst reading through any remedy which has both these symptoms check for the rest of the symptoms – the correct remedy should also be *anxious, restless* and *fearful*, it will not be a dull, indifferent kind of remedy. It should also be better for fresh air and worse in a warm, stuffy room, worse for touch and for noise. Each symptom you check out should considerably narrow down your choice of remedy and you should arrive at one remedy which is most similar to the whole symptom picture. If two or more remedies seem to fit, choose the remedy which is the *most similar*. Your symptom analysis grid will help you greatly in the task of recognizing the most similar remedy.

Case example 1

A child comes home from school and then goes out to ride on his bicycle. There is a cold, dry wind blowing and the child is insufficiently dressed for the weather. A couple of hours later, on being put to bed in his centrally heated bedroom, he suddenly says he feels unwell. He is hot, his head aches, he obviously has a temperature and he is suddenly sick. Whilst being cleaned up he complains every time he is touched. He asks to have the window opened and says fresh air makes him feel a bit better. He keeps tossing and turning restlessly and complaining of aches and pains. He complains that there is a bitter taste in his mouth and his throat feels sore. He asks for a drink of cold water, drinks it thirstily and soon wants more. The aches and pains seem to be making him anxious and restless, and with the sudden onset of a very painful earache the child actually becomes really fearful. Although he is usually quite fearful of the dark he asks to have the light off as it makes his headache worse. He asks people to be quiet because the noise irritates him and makes his head and ears ache worse. The music from a radio in the next room makes him irritable.

Here we have a jumble of symptoms as they actually present themselves. Firstly we make a list of the presenting symptoms.

Symptoms appear suddenly: came on after exposure to cold, dry wind; vomiting; high temperature; headache < light, < noise; generally < touch; generally > fresh air; generally < warm, stuffy room; restlessness; bitter taste in the mouth; very thirsty for cold water; anxious, fearful; sore throat; generally < noise and < music.

Now, to make the symptom picture even clearer we will put the symptoms into their appropriate categories. This helps us to evaluate the symptoms, and also to compare them with remedies at a glance. Remember to underline any characteristic symptoms for ease of reference – these may lead you directly to the appropriate remedy or leave you with only a few from which to choose.

Abbreviations: worse = < better = >

Mode of onset:	Sudden
Possible cause:	Exposure to cold, dry windy weather
Mental/Emotional:	Restless, anxious, fearful
General:	Very thirsty for cold water; vomiting, hot
Particular:	Headache, sore throat, bitter taste, earache
Modalities	
Mental/Emotional:	None
General:	< Warm stuffy room < touch < music < noise > fresh air
Particular:	Headache < light < noise; earache < noise

The symptoms of vomiting, sore throat and high temperature

are common symptoms and could be found in many remedies. More information would be needed about these symptoms for them to be useful in narrowing down the remedy selection. The mental/emotional symptoms are characteristic of only a few remedies, and so are of more importance.

Enter the symptoms into your photocopied symptom analysis grid and systematically search through your remedies, filling in the grid as shown in Example A, page 44.

Case example 2

It is a warm, wet morning in spring. A child wakes up feeling unwell and apathetic; he does not want to eat all his breakfast. He goes out to play in the garden but he seems unusually tired and lethargic. At dinner he attempts to eat a little and then is sick. He goes to lie down and after a little while he complains of a headache. He says his arms and legs feel tired and heavy. He just wants to lie down quietly and not be disturbed. His mouth is dry; his mother offers him a drink but he says he is not thirsty, he does not want anything. His eyes look dull and heavy and his face gradually becomes a dull, dusky pink. His skin feels warm and moist. Mildness of temperament. He wants to spend a penny and on sitting up he feels dizzy. On returning from the loo, after voiding a large quantity of clear urine, he says his head feels a bit better and so he gets up for a while, looking a bit brighter. However, after a short time he feels sick and dizzy and wants to go and lie down quietly again. He has a sensation of shivers up and down the spine. When the other children come into the bedroom he is irritated by their noise and presence and asks them to leave him alone.

Presenting symptoms: Symptoms came on slowly and gradually; came on in warm, wet weather; loss of appetite; tiredness; vomiting; headache ameliorated by profuse urination; feels better lying down; feels worse sitting up; limbs feel heavy and weary; mouth dry with no thirst; face dull, dusky pink; skin warm, moist; eyes heavy and dull; mildness of temperament – asks for nothing; irritation on being disturbed; wants to be left alone; sensation of shivers up and down the spine; dullness; drowsiness; heaviness;

weariness; indifference; generally better after profuse urination; dizziness on sitting up.

Now we put these symptoms into their appropriate categories:

Mode of onset:	Came on slowly and gradually
Possible cause:	Unknown. The weather is warm and wet but we cannot be sure if it caused the disturbance in the child, but keep it in mind
Mental/emotional:	Indifference, desire to be left alone, apathetic
General:	Heaviness, weariness drowsiness, thirstless (with a dry mouth), dizziness (on sitting up), shivers, vomiting, loss of appetite
Particular:	Eyes – heavy, dull; Limbs – heavy, tired; Mouth – dry; Face – dull, dusky pink; Skin – warm, moist; Headache
Modalities	
Mental/emotional:	None
General:	> Lying down, < sitting up
Particular:	Headache > urination

Now enter the most characteristic, striking or unusual symptoms, including modalities, into an analysis grid and then search systematically through your remedy pictures, filling in the grid as previously shown.

There is no need to use every symptom in your cases. Ten symptoms are quite adequate, though you can use more or less as required. If you use more you will have to adjust your grid to accommodate the extra symptoms.

Case example 3

A gardener comes indoors one evening, after a hard day's work out in the hot sun. He looks very tired and red-faced. He complains of a terrible headache, which he says has been getting progressively worse since mid-morning. He is very irritable and very worried about the work that he should have completed, but could not because the headache was becoming so bad. His throat becomes sore and so his wife looks at it and sees that it is very red. He says that it feels sore and dry. He has a bit of a temperature; he feels hot and dry to the touch. He is impatient for something to be done to make him feel better quickly so that he can get some more work done. His wife decides to try a homoeopathic remedy for him and begins to ask him some questions.

Answering questions makes him very irritable – he says thinking makes his head throb even more. He is extremely thirsty and drinks down a glass of water very quickly. His wife presses his forehead with her hand to see if the pressure will help him and he says this relieves the pain quite a lot. He is very tired and goes to lie down in a darkish room. He presses the painful part into the pillow and this gives him some relief. He says he feels better from lying down and keeping still; he says that moving around increases the suffering. He is very thirsty and sits up to drink another glass of water; sitting up makes him feel dizzy and faint. He is very hot and worse for being in a warm, stuffy room so asks to have the window open and feels a little better for cool fresh air.

Presenting symptoms: Symptoms came on gradually; came on in hot sun; headache, throbbing, < movement, < thinking, > pressure; impatient; irritable; worries about his work; throat – red, sore, dry; temperature; hot and dry; very thirsty for long, cold drinks of water; > from keeping still; < from movement; > from lying down; < from warm, stuffy room; > from fresh air; < from sitting up (feels dizzy and faint).

Now put these symptoms into their appropriate categories. Reference to examples 1 and 2 will give you the idea of how to do this. Now, enter the symptoms into the analysis grid and work out the most appropriate remedy.

8. Guidelines to Taking the Remedies

Homoeopathic remedies are generally used in the form of tiny pills called pillules. One pillule should be placed, dry, under the tongue and allowed to dissolve. It is also permissible to dissolve the remedy in a small tumblerful of water and take two teaspoonsful at the required intervals. *Tinctures should never be taken internally*. Apply externally as advised.

Timing of the doses

The frequency of repetition of the doses is dependent on the acuteness of the patient's condition. It is a good idea to allow half an hour to one hour between doses at first, lengthening the intervals to several hours between doses as benefit to the patient becomes apparent.

Generally, the more acute the case, the closer the doses need to be. In *very* acute cases, 15 minutes may be adequate time to wait before reconsidering your remedy selection.

Number of doses

Usually you will find that two or three doses of the correctly chosen remedy are sufficient to help the patient recover. Always *stop* the remedy doses as soon as an improvement is noticed. Give the remedy time to complete its action.

Always watch the patient's response to the remedy given and wait for the signs which indicate your next course of action – whether this is to repeat the same remedy, make a new remedy selection or do nothing because the patient needs no more treatment.

What to do if a new symptom picture occurs

Some conditions, such as colds, measles, etc. go through several well-defined stages. At each stage a new remedy may be called for, always basing your choice on the picture presented by the patient and not on the common symptoms of the diagnosed condition.

Results of the correct remedy selection

If the chosen remedy is homoeopathic to the patient, that is, if it is truly the most similar in its symptom picture to the symptom picture of the patient, the patient will experience a greater sense of well-being, including a lifting of spirits, followed by an alleviation of all unpleasant symptoms. Or they may fall into a peaceful sleep and awake feeling better all round. These are two common reactions to the correctly selected remedy.

Natural response of the body

The effect of the correct remedy prescription is to accelerate the natural healing abilities and responses of the body. It stimulates the same mechanism which is already at work within the body, dealing with the illness, thus enhancing the effort. This can, occasionally, *temporarily* aggravate the presenting symptoms, as the body's defences work more effectively to restore order to the patient. Sometimes, this may cause the patient's temperature to rise slightly before falling, or cause the nauseous patient to vomit before being relieved, or the itching to increase before subsiding. This exacerbation of symptoms is not always noticeable in acute cases, as the symptoms are already at a high pitch, However, if it does occur, wait for the aggravation to subside before re-evaluating the position.

However, always use your common sense. Remember that the chosen remedy may be wrong and the dis-ease process may simply be following its course. If a temperature rises too high or the situation is otherwise disturbing, *always* call professional help.

Reconsidering your remedy selection if no improvement

The wrongly chosen medicine appears to have no effect, one way or the other, on the patient. If there is no definite improvement in the patient after two or three doses of the seemingly correct remedy, then it should be discontinued, the case re-evaluated and a more appropriate remedy given.

In the early days of your acquaintance with homoeopathy it is quite often necessary to have to try several remedies before finding the correct one. This is quite safe to do providing you stick to the low potency recommended. As you grow in experience and confidence you are more likely to find the correct remedy sooner. However, do not give two remedies together; always give one remedy time to act before considering your next move.

Be observant

In an acute illness, much energy is needed by the body to establish recovery. The homoeopathic prescriber should be aware of the rise and fall of the patient's vitality and intensity of symptoms, as this will give indications for repeating or waiting. As a general rule, if the patient appears better in themselves, experiences an increased sense of well-being, is calm and coherent, or is simply sleeping peacefully, you can take this to be an improvement.

Part Three

9. The Remedy Pictures

Introduction to the remedy pictures

We have called the descriptions of the remedies 'pictures', as they evoke in the mind of the reader an image. Each remedy picture has its own personality with its own way of expressing itself, just as all people do. To match the remedy picture with the individual's symptom picture is one of the objectives of the homoeopathic prescriber.

A note of caution

Be aware that some symptom complexes, if taken in isolation, may relate to conditions which could be diagnosed by a doctor as requiring immediate medical attention. In any situation where you would normally call your doctor or health professional, do so. You may of course prescribe an appropriate homoeopathic remedy while you wait for help to arrive. This is the safe way to approach a medical situation that you are not sure of.

It is not the aim of this book to encourage individuals to tackle situations which require professional medical attention. Use the remedies to cope with the more manageable conditions that occur from time to time in every home. With practice you will realize the potential that homoeopathy holds for promoting harmony and health for the whole family. Do not allow self-importance to prevent you from asking for help from an appropriate source if you have need of it.

Remedy layout and language

The remedies are laid out for ease of reference in the language of symptoms as expressed by the provers. The picture attempts to express the essence of the remedies, noting characteristic, general, mental and emotional aspects followed by sections relating to the particular spheres over which each remedy has the greatest influence. The remedy pictures, even in the condensed form in which they appear here, cover far more than you will ever probably require. This has been done in an attempt to maintain the essence of the remedies. Avoid thinking in absolutes and consider the symptoms in degrees of intensity.

For example, on looking through Belladonna, you may think it sounds quite a desperate case. In its entirety indeed it is. And yet it is one of the most widely used remedies, particularly in children suffering from acute ailments which exhibit a likeness to the Belladonna symptom picture in its various forms and degrees of intensity. Remember, nobody would have all the symptoms of a remedy. However, the remedy chosen should cover most of the ones they do have.

Contradictions

It is interesting to note that apparent contradictions appear in some remedies. This simply indicates that individual provers have experienced opposite states from the same remedy. As long as you pay attention to the totality of the case and are able to match it within a remedy picture, this should not cause you problems.

Aconite

Aconitum Napellus

The picture – mentals and generals

The action of Aconite is sudden, short and painful. It is suitable in the first stage of an acute condition which comes on suddenly. Aconite is anxious, restless, fearful and tense. There may be irritability and impatience. The Aconite causation is very characteristic. The most common causes are:

1. becoming chilled, especially after exposure to cold, dry winds;
2. sudden shock or fright;
3. a soaking;
4. extreme heat.

It is also useful after injuries, operations or difficulties in childbirth where there has been fright or shock, or after anger. A person requiring Aconite will generally produce symptoms the same day of the exposure. The symptoms come on suddenly. Aconite should be given early, whilst the symptoms are still intense.

Aconite is known as one of the nursery remedies, together with Belladonna and Chamomilla. This trio are also sometimes called the ABC remedies as they are very often useful for the first stages of acute illness which children are often prone to. It is generally suited to strong, rosy individuals who tend to sudden acute storms of illness which are soon over. There is generally restlessness and sleeplessness with tossing about. There is fear and panic in this remedy and sometimes fear of death. Very useful for women who become panic stricken and fearful during labour. The pains are insupportable and the Aconite patient often makes a lot of noise and holds the painful part. The pain and fear can be evident in the facial expression. It is often useful in fevers where the patient is burning hot and dry, red and tense. The senses are heightened and they are especially sensitive to noise, light and touch. The pains are usually worse during the evening and at night. They are worse in a stuffy room and desire cool, fresh, open air. Aconite is hot and dry and thirsty for cold water. Sometimes, everything can taste bitter except water. It is useful in sudden nosebleeds when the blood is bright red, particularly when accompanied by anxiety or even panic. There can be agonizing and restlessness from fear and from pain. Threatened abortion from fright. Pains may be accompanied by sensations of numbness or tingling.

Particular spheres of usefulness

Head: Aches with heat, heaviness, burning, fullness.
Face: Hot and dry, neuralgic pains, can be accompanied by numbness or tingling. One cheek red, other pale.
Eyes: Hot and dry, red and swollen lids.
Teeth: Insupportable pain, worse from cold draughts with great thirst for cold water.
Throat: Sore, hot, dry, red, constricted, tingling, burning, smarting.
Chest: Cough – short, dry, croupy, worse on inspiration and at night, with sensation of suffocation, hard, nothing coughed up except a little watery mucus. Dry, loud, spasmodic, wakes him from sleep with anxiety and panic, tightness of chest.
Colds: From exposure to cold, dry winds, with fever, thirst for cold water, headache and sleeplessness.
Abdomen: Hot, tense, distended, sensitive to touch, cutting pains, colic, watery diarrhoea or greenish like chopped spinach.
Urinary: Scanty, hot, painful, suppressed. Retention or suppression of urine in newborn babies. Retention from chill, cold, fright, shock with anxiety and restlessness, cutting, tearing, burning pains, thirst.
Heart: Palpitations, rapid, full, bounding pulse with awful anxiety, heat and thirst.
Sleep: Sleeplessness with tossing about, fear, anguish, from chill, shock, fright, after operations.
Fever: Chills alternating with dry, burning heat, must uncover. Chills with shivering, creeping sensations. Skin hot, dry, burning or as if ice-water on it. Thirst for long drinks. Likes to be sponged down with cool water. Fever with tossing about and restlessness.
Modalities: *Worse from*: fright, shock, cold winds, cold, dry weather, night, light, touch, noise, music, warm, stuffy rooms, dentition.
Better from: Open air, warm sweating.

Apis mellifica

The Sting of the Honey Bee

The picture – mentals and generals

The effects of a bee sting – shiny, rosy-red, watery swellings: burning, prickling, itching, stinging sensations. Stinging pains, as if hot needles were sticking in. Sudden pains give rise to sudden, piercing shrieks, which even interrupt sleep. Apis has a marked effect on the coverings of the organism – skin, mucous membranes. It particularly affects the face, eyes, throat and ovaries. It affects mainly the right side. Swellings puffy, watery, looking like puffy bags of water. The symptoms develop with violence and rapidity. Burning, smarting and itching. The Apis patient is made much worse from heat – worse in a warm room, worse from sitting near the fire, worse from a hot bath. Heat is one of the worst things for an Apis patient and intensely aggravates them. They are also generally worse on waking, after sleep. Apis patients are extremely sensitive to touch. Tremblings and twitchings. Apis patients are extremely restless, fidgety and depressed, though they often slide gradually into a state of apathy and stupor. Can move from irritability to apathy. Weepy for no reason. Inability to concentrate the mind on attempting to study. Ill effects of shocks, fright, grief, vexation, jealousy, suppressed eruptions. Generally much aggravated by heat and ameliorated by cool. Nervous and hysterical conditions. Fussy and fidgety. Jealous and suspicious. Awkward, restless and irritable. Scanty or suppressed urination. An increased flow of urine is often a sign that Apis has begun a favourable action. Thirstlessness – drinks little. Retention of urine in babies.

Particular spheres of usefulness

Head: Pains which are worse from warmth and better from cool and from pressure.

Eyes: Swelling of the eyelids, watery, puffy, rosy-red swellings as if full of water, under the eyes. Burning, stinging, itching.

Face: Watery swellings with smarting, burning sensations.

Mouth: Tongue feels burnt, sore; grinding of the teeth.

Throat: Inflamed, red, swollen; uvula swollen, red and glistening, hanging down like a large, semi-transparent bag of water. Stinging, burning pains which are ameliorated by cold drinks. Throat sore, worse swallowing solids. Sense of constriction in throat.

Respiration: Air hunger. Breathing hurried and difficult. Chest sore. Pain from coughing. Suffocating sensations. Cannot bear anything about the throat.

Abdomen: Tight and distended; very sensitive to pressure. Sensation as though something would break if too much effort were made on straining at stool. Diarrhoea with sensation as though anus remained open.

Urinary: Burning, stinging, smarting pains. Urine burning, scanty, highly coloured. Retention or suppression. Retention in newborn babies. Stinging pains, with thirstlessness, worse from heat. An increased flow of urine is an indication that Apis has begun a favourable action.

Female: Burning, stinging pains in ovaries, right side more affected. Stinging pains in breasts. Menses suppressed or scanty with headaches and faintness.

Skin: Rosy-red, watery swellings. Scarlet eruptions. Burning, stinging, itching, smarting.

Heart: Palpitations.

Fever: Thirstlessness during the sweat: thirst may or may not be present during the heat; thirst during the chill. Chills alternate with heat. Sweat breaks out and dries up frequently.

Modalities: *Worse from*: Heat in any form, hot drinks, hot rooms, hot baths, on waking from sleep, from pressure (except head, which is better from pressure), lying down, suppressed eruptions. Touch.

Better from: Cold air, cold bathing, motion, sitting erect, slight expectoration.

Arsenicum album

Arsenic

The picture – mentals and generals

Arsenicum is particularly suited to patients who are anxious, restless and fearful, nervous, highly strung, easily startled and frightened, easily irritated, can be impatient. Exacting, fastidious people who are easily disturbed by any disorder in their surroundings. There is great restlessness, the patient must be constantly on the move, driven by the tremendous mental anxiety, despite rapid weakness and exhaustion. There is often a nightly aggravation, around midnight and shortly after midnight. The characteristic pains of Arsenicum are burning, yet strangely are ameliorated by heat. Arsenicum is an extremely chilly patient who likes to be covered up warmly up to the neck, yet likes the head to be cool, in a breeze of fresh air. The patient is full of anxiety and dread. There is anxiety when alone, in the evening and when going to bed, which drives him out of the bed. Despite the weakness and lack of vitality, the Arsenicum patient cannot rest if their surroundings are not in order. Arsenicum can be a methodical, fault-finding, fussy patient. Arsenicum is often indicated for the bad effects of eating spoiled foods, especially bad meat, also bad effects from eating watery fruits and vegetables. Diarrhoea and vomiting, often simultaneous, accompanied by sudden intense weakness, forcing them to lie down. There may be an unquenchable thirst for cold water, which may be vomited immediately. Burning stomach pains which are sometimes ameliorated by warm water. Takes small sips, little and often. In digestive upsets and nausea they cannot bear the sight, smell or sometimes even the thought of food. The discharges are usually thin and watery and excoriating, making the surrounding parts sore.

Particular spheres of usefulness

Head: Congestive headaches better from cold water and cool fresh air; with restlessness, head in constant motion. Sick headaches with nausea and vomiting and thirst for little and often.

Colds: Thin, watery, excoriating discharge. Violent sneezing. Nose stopped up. Colds begin in nose and descend to chest. Worse from draughts and change of weather.

Face: Watery, puffy swellings, particularly around the eyes.

Respiration: Shortness of breath. Sensation of suffocation with anguish, unable to lie down, must sit up; worse at night, from windy weather, from heat of room, from being fatigued, from being angry, from laughing, from movement; better from cold, fresh air; with anxious face, covered in cold sweat; anxious, wheezy respiration.

Cough: Dry, hacking cough; little or no expectoration; worse around midnight. Very chilly. Wheezy breathing. Patient chilly, exhausted, restless and anxious.

Stomach: Loss of appetite, cannot bear sight, smell or even thought of food. Desire for cold water, acids, sour things, coffee, brandy, milk. Aversion to sweets, fats, meat. Unquenchable thirst, drinks small sips often. Desires ice-cold water which is vomited immediately. Often better for warm water. Nausea, retching, vomiting and purging. Ill effects of spoiled foods, bad meat, watery fruits and vegetables. Anxiety felt in the pit of stomach.

Abdomen: Colicky pains with vomiting, diarrhoea and weakness. Gnawing, burning pains with anxiety, incredible restlessness and full of despair. Diarrhoea with weakness which necessitates lying down, worse from watery fruits and cold drinks. Piles, burning, better from warm applications.

Neck/back: Drawing pains in back necessitating lying down. Weakness, as if bruised, in small of back.

Extremities: Watery swellings in feet. Tinglings in fingers. Uneasiness of lower limbs – must move them constantly. Thick skin on soles of feet.

Skin: Dry and rough. Ulceration with offensive discharges. Hot, itching and burning. Pale and puffy watery swellings, inflammations. Burning itchiness – they scratch till it bleeds.

Sleep: Restless and anxious. Sleeplessness, tossing and turning with anguish after midnight. Starting with general fright and uneasiness during sleep. Lies with head held high.

Fever: Coldness. Skin dry, like parchment. During the chill, no thirst except for warm drinks; during heat, little and often; cold during the sweat, great thirst for large quantities. Burning, internal heat with external coldness. Cold sweats. Exhaustion and prostration. Restlessness and anxiety. Worst time is midnight till 3am.

Modalities: *Worse from*: Night, midnight and shortly after, cold air, cold foods, watery fruits and vegetables, spoiled food, bad meat, suppressed eruptions, seashore, exertion.

Better from: Heat (warm applications, food, drinks), lying with head held high, warm wraps, open air, sweating.

Belladonna

Deadly Nightshade

The picture – mentals and generals

Belladonna is bright red, burning hot, dry and throbbing. Symptoms appear suddenly and disappear just as suddenly. Belladonna comes on with acuteness, violence and intensity. The sweat appears and disappears suddenly. Congestions to the head. Hot head with cold hands and feet. Complaints, particularly headaches, after exposure to the hot sun. Sudden, intense fevers. Patient almost in a stupor. Semi-stupor. Half-awake, half-asleep. Delirium with all sorts of strange imaginations and fears. Sees monsters and faces. Violent delirium, restlessness. Belladonna is particularly suitable for people who are vigorous and good-humoured when well, but become violent when sick. They can be wild, bad-tempered, irritable, furious. The predominant emotion of Belladonna is anger. They make a lot of noise and let everyone know they are suffering. Extremely oversensitive. Sensitive to the pain, and to noise, light, pressure and touch. Cannot bear touch to the head. Cannot stand cold applications. Sudden intense fevers with bright red face, burning, radiating heat. In extreme cases they bite, strike and tear things. Wild expression. Wild staring eyes with big pupils. Throbbing pains. Spasms are also characteristic of Belladonna, ranging from mild little twitchings to the most violent convulsions. Right-sided symptoms are most usual. Bright red streaks radiating outwards. Craves lemonade. Talks fast. Heat and swellings. Localized inflammations. Impatience.

Particular spheres of usefulness

Head: Throbbing, pulsating pains. Congestions to the head with heat. Sensitive to draughts and cold air, to washing hair, to having the hair touched. Sunstroke and headaches from exposure to heat of the sun. Rubbing of head on to pillow. Dizziness from rising or stooping.

Eyes: Hot and burning. Lids sore, heavy, red. Very sensitive to light. Pupils dilated. Eyes staring. Bloodshot.

Throat: Inflamed, swollen, dry, hot and bright red. Difficulty swallowing from constriction or spasm. Often worse on the right side.

Abdomen: Hot and inflamed, tender and distended and painful. Pain worse from the slightest jarring. Worse right side. (*Beware*: this symptom complex may indicate appendicitis, so call doctor.) Violent intense colic. Sudden pains. Constipation. Fruitless urging. Spasmodic contractions.

Cough: Dry cough from tickling and burning sensations. Violent bouts of coughing. Feels as if head would burst. Child cries before coughing attack starts. As soon as the violent coughing has raised some mucus there is peace and the coughing stops. As

	the throat grows drier the tickling starts again, and then the spasmodic coughing. Spasms, gagging and whooping.
Female:	Menses of bright red, hot blood, profuse. Cramping and bearing down pains during menses, worse right side, worse lying down, better standing and sitting erect. Red streaks radiating outwards from nipples.
Extremities:	Joints red, shiny, hot, swollen, better from heat, worse cold.
Skin:	Bright red, dry, hot, shiny. Streaks of radiating redness.
Sleep:	Sees horrible visions on closing the eyes. Moans and twitches during sleep.
Modalities:	*Worse from:* Heat of sun, washing head. Light, noise, jarring, touch, company, pressure, motion, looking at shining objects or running water. *Better from:* Light covering, bending backward, standing, leaning head against something.

Bryonia

Wild Hops

The picture – mentals and generals

Bryonia is a remedy of short-lasting, acute action, the symptoms develop slowly over the course of a few hours to a few days, like Gelsemium. The chief characteristic symptom of Bryonia is its exceptional sensitivity to motion of any kind – physical or mental. Even the motion of the eyes increases their suffering. Anything which compels them to think or move worsens them. Often they will not answer questions because the effort of being forced to think aggravates them. With their great sensitivity to motion Bryonia are ameliorated by pressure – they will tend to lie on the painful part to keep it still. (Belladonna will lie only on the side which is not painful as they are so sensitive to the slightest pressure.) The characteristic pains of Bryonia are sticking and stitching. Sticking and stitching pains worse from motion. Everywhere there is dryness, the lips are parched and dry. The stools are dry and hard, hence a greatly used remedy in constipation. There is a great thirst for long cold drinks which they will swig down in one go. They feel much worse in a hot, stuffy atmosphere and better from cool air. They feel worse from sitting up – sick, dizzy and faint. They feel restless but do not tend to move much because of the aggravation it causes them. Bryonia is very useful in complaints coming on after humiliation and anger, from overeating, from suppressed eruptions and discharges. Bryonia is irritable, touchy, impatient and obsessed with work. In mild delirium the patient is obsessed with the idea of wanting to go home (even if they are home) to go and get on with their work. Non-appearance or slow development of rashes or eruptions in eruptive dis-eases. The patient is irritable, dry and touchy. Anxiety about the future. Wants to be left alone. Averse to talking. Capricious.

Particular spheres of usefulness

Head: Dizzy and faint on raising up the head, and when stooping. Bursting, throbbing and stitching headaches, worse for motion, stooping, coughing, etc. Must lie down and keep absolutely still.

Face: Dark, purply red, or pale yellow, earth coloured. Lips dry, cracked.

Mouth: Dryness of mouth, tongue and throat. Coated tongue. Excessive thirst for cold drinks.

Cough: Dry, hacking cough, worse after eating and drinking, must sit up. Cough worse for deep breathing, night, warm room. Child kicks covers off. With cough, stitching pains in the chest and must support chest with hand. Constant desire to take a deep breath, which then causes coughing and shooting, stitching pains in the chest. Breathing quick, difficult and anxious. Cough excited by tickling in the throat. Great thirst. Dry spasmodic cough with gagging and vomiting. Breathing short and rapid and deep breathing is painful.

Stomach:	Thirst for cold water. Nausea on rising up. Acid or bitter risings after eating. Pressure, as of a stone on stomach, after eating. Stomach sensitive to touch. Complaints after over-eating, e.g. children who have overindulged at parties.
Abdomen:	Dryness. Constipation – stools hard and dry. Constipation of tourists.
Female:	Suppression of the menses with nosebleed or headache.
Extremities:	Hot, swollen red joints, worse for least motion. Sticking, stitching, tearing pains.
Skin:	Burning, prickling.
Fever:	With great thirst. Lies perfectly still. Worse for motion. Irritable.
Modalities:	*Worse from*: Least motion, raising up, stooping, coughing, deep breathing, heat, eating, touch. *Better from*: Rest, cool air, cold drinks, lying on painful part, quiet, pressure.

Calcarea carbonica

Carbonate of Lime, Middle Layer of Oyster Shell

The picture – mentals and generals

Calcarea is most suitable to persons who are pale, heavy, very sensitive, slow in movement and sweat easily. They are extremely chilly and sensitive to cold, damp air. They take cold easily and it often goes to the chest. They are easily exhausted. Lacking in endurance. They are worse from exertion – worse from ascending stairs, particularly in respiratory troubles. Tendency to easy and profuse perspiration. Sweats on the head and neck at night, wetting the pillow all around. The feet are cold and damp. The hands are cold and clammy. It is very often indicated in children. Chubby, mischievous children with sweaty heads. Calcarea will sit for long periods doing nothing or playing with the fingers. They are often slow to walk, slow to grow teeth, fontanelles slow to close. There is easy sweating on exertion. The typical Calcarea child is often obstinate, mischievous and self-willed. Craving for cold things, particularly ice-cream. Craving for eggs, particularly soft-boiled eggs. Calcarea is full of fears and anxieties. Sensitive to hearing horrible stories, sensitive to reprimands, sensitive to being looked at – think people are laughing at them. They can be irritable and impatient. They can see visions and faces on closing the eyes at night. Very fearful and easily frightened. Fearful of the dark. Cannot rest. Cannot go to sleep so that the mind and body rests. Horrible dreams, disturbing sleep. Awake for a large part of the night. Awakes from bad dreams in fright. Child grinds the teeth during sleep, making chewing and swallowing motions during sleep. Tendency to cramps, especially in calves when in bed at night. Worse from cold, damp air, draughts and cold bathing. Weakness, easily exhausted mentally, as well as physically. Dwells on insignificant matters, rambles on about them. Easily mesmerized, likes to be mesmerized. Easily startled by noise. Often indicated during dentition when teeth are late to come through or come through with great attendant difficulties. Tendency to easy strains and sprains. Cannot bear to be the centre of attention. Sensitive to atmospheres.

Particular spheres of usefulness

Head: Easy and profuse sweat on head and neck at night, icy-cold sensation on top of head, or burning heat. Aches worse from wind, better on closing eyes, better for pressure. Aches from overlifting, from muscular strains. Vertigo, worse ascending.

Eyes: Sensitive to light, easy watering in open air, dimness of sight, particularly after reading or concentrating. Easy fatigue from exertion.

Face: Upper lip cracked and swollen. Swollen, painful, inflamed glands.

Colds: Sensitive to cold and damp. Worse from cold air, working in cold water, cold bathing, cold, damp weather. Also sensitive to heat of sun. Sweats easily. Offensive, thick, yellow discharge, accumulation of thick crusts in nose. Nose becomes stopped up at night. Colds and catarrhs of children during teething. Inflamed tonsils. Swollen glands.

Cough: Tickling cough excited by sensation of dust in throat, easily out of breath particularly on exertion and when ascending stairs. Habit cough. Takes cold easily. Rattling of mucus, chest painfully sensitive to touch and on inspiration.

Stomach: Desires ice-cream, salt, sweets, soft-boiled eggs, raw foods such as raw potatoes, indigestible things such as chalk, coal. Aversion to meat and hot foods. Great thirst for cold drinks. Stomach swollen and large and painful on pressure. Sour vomiting. Sour eructations, vomiting of sour milk, curds.

Abdomen: Enlarged and hard, sensations of coldness, swollen, painful glands. Chalky-white stools.

Extremities: Feet cold and damp, hands cold and clammy. Tends to cramps in calves, especially at night. Soles of feet burning hot in bed at night. Limbs go to sleep whilst sitting, stiffness in joints on beginning to move. Stiffness worse from working in water. Swollen joints. Easy spraining and straining. Weakness. Numbness. Stiffness.

Back: Pain in back as if sprained, causing difficulty in rising from seat.

Skin: Cold skin. Cold profuse sweat. Clammy. Wounds take a long time to heal. Ulcerations.

Modalities: *Worse from*: Cold air, cold bathing, exertion, ascending, eye strain, milk, pressure of clothes, full moon, teething.
Better from: dry weather, rubbing, after breakfast.

Carbo vegetabilis

Wood Charcoal

The picture – mentals and generals

Carbo veg. in its crude state has deodorant and antiseptic properties, which are greatly increased when it is potentized.

It is a very useful remedy in states of absolute collapse, with cold breath, cold sweat and weak pulse, and can be given whilst waiting for help to arrive. Surprisingly, considering all this coldness, the Carbo veg. patient wants cold air, wants to be fanned, sometimes wants cold water. There is a strong desire for fresh air, with absolute weakness. Carbo veg. patients have a sensation of overfullness, heaviness, bloatedness. Everything seems to be swollen, relaxed and puffed. Blueness, coldness and sluggishness. The patient feels so puffed and overfull that he just wants to lie down. Carbo veg. has earned a reputation as a reviver in states of complete collapse – the remedy dissolved in a small quantity of water and the lips and mouth frequently moistened with the solution. Digestive complaints are another sphere of usefulness of Carbo veg. It is one of the most flatulent of remedies. Sluggish digestion, food turns to gas. The discomfort is relieved, temporarily, by loud, rancid belching. Sluggishness and disorder of the digestive system, brought on by years of feeding on rich and fatty foods, sweets, pies and puddings. Mentally slow, lazy, sluggish, indifferent. Lack of reaction. Lack of recuperation. Never been really well since a previous illness or shock. Internal burning and external coldness. Over-relaxed. Slow repair. Septic conditions. Ulcerations. Purpled, mottled appearance of the skin. Generally indifferent. Averse to darkness and fearful of ghosts.

Particular spheres of usefulness

Head: Dull, heavy ache, worse from over-indulgence, pressure, lying, becoming overheated.

Face: Pale, pinched, cold, bluish, cold sweat.

Stomach: Slow digestion. Food turns to gas. Loud, rancid eructations, which relieve temporarily. Desire for salt, sweets, coffee, which makes them sick. Averse to milk, meat. Heavy, full, sleepy after eating. Face flushes easily after wine.

Abdomen: Affects mainly upper part of abdomen. Pain, distension, flatulence. Flatulent colic. Cannot bear any pressure (of clothing, etc.). Diarrhoea from bad food with distension. Piles, bluish, burning, pain after stools.

Cough/ respiration: Hoarseness, worse evenings, worse warm, wet, damp air. Cough spasmodic, dry, hard, rough, hollow, whooping; with blue face; with retching, gagging and vomiting. Breath cold, yet wants cold air; must be fanned. Cough worse evenings, movement, walking in open air, cold wet weather, change of temperature from warm to cold, after lying, after eating and drinking. Desires to take a deep breath Shortness of breath and difficulty in breathing. Wheezy breathing with rattling of mucus on chest. Pain in chest after cough.

Fever: Internal burning heat with external coldness. Cold skin, cold sweat.

Modalities: *Worse from*: Warmth, previous exhausting illness, rich foods, fatty foods, butter, coffee, milk, warm, damp, pressure of clothes.
Better from: Eructations, cold air, being fanned.

Chamomilla

German Chamomile

The picture – mentals and generals

Chamomilla is chiefly famous for its anger and oversensitivity, particularly to pain. It is not suited to those who bear their pain with calmness and patience. Its action is acute, sudden and short-lasting. It is usually associated with teething babies, but although it is one of the chief nursery remedies for babies and children, it is useful for anyone where the characteristic symptoms are present. Chamomilla is sometimes known as the *can't bear it* remedy. Cannot bear the pain, everything is unendurable. Chamomilla is emotional, temperamental, oversensitive, badtempered, irritable and demanding. Chamomilla babies will hold out their little hands for first one thing then push it away and cry for something else, never satisfied. They are extremely restless, want to be carried about and amused. When older they demand things, then refuse them, or complain about them when offered. They are very restless, must be moving about with the pains. They demand that someone **do something**. Chamomilla is thirsty, hot and numb. They get too hot in bed, cannot bear staying in bed and are driven out of it by their discomfort. Their feet burn in bed and they must stick them out of the covers to cool them. Worse during the evening and night. Hot clammy sweat on the forehead and scalp. A cross, complaining patient. Restlessness. One cheek hot and red, the other cold and pale. Pains generally better from warmth, except teeth pains which are worse for warmth, better for cold water. Symptoms coming on after anger and indignation. Cough, colic, diarrhoea, any condition after anger. Hot sweat. Child stiffens out. Often useful in teething babies, where the teething is accompanied by crossness, restlessness, diarrhoea, sweaty head and is only pacified by being carried constantly.

Particular spheres of usefulness

Head: Throbbing headache, often one-sided. Hot clammy sweat on forehead and scalp, wetting the hair.

Face: One cheek brilliant red and hot, the other pale and cool.

Ears: Earache better from warmth. Sensitive to cold air.

Teeth: Toothache worse from warm drinks, worse from coffee. Frantic with the pain. Teething babies driven to distraction.

Cough: Hard, dry, hacking cough, worse at night, coughs in sleep without waking. Dry, tickling cough. Coughing bouts as a result of anger and indignation. Rattling of mucus on chest. Suffocating cough.

Stomach: Bitter bilious vomiting. Pressive pain. Worse from coffee. Great thirst for cold water. Foul eructations like bad eggs.

Abdomen: Cutting, windy, colic, after anger, with red cheeks and hot perspiration. Better from warm applications. Distended abdomen. Diarrhoea during dentition, diarrhoea from anger. Diarrhoea sour, grass green or yellow, slimy or watery. Particularly suitable in teething babies who are extremely irritable and cross, must be carried.

Extremities: Violent rheumatic pains compelling patient to get out of bed at night and walk around. Burning of soles of feet at night – must stick them out of the bed. Numbness accompanying pain. Cannot bear the pain.

Female: Intolerable labour pains. Unendurable after pains. Menstrual colic driving her to distraction. Women who become capricious, bad tempered and irritable before menses. Often useful in pregnancy and labour when the characteristic symptoms are present, cross and complaining.

Skin: Red rashes of babies and nursing mothers from anger and indignation. Yellowness particularly following anger.

Sleep: Restlessness, sleepless from abuse of coffee, pain killers and sleeping tablets.

Fever: One part cold, another part hot, alternately chilly and hot, sweats on head, hot and clammy sweat. Great thirst during fever.

Modalities: *Worse from:* Anger, teething, coffee, stimulants, pain killers, sleeping pills, night 9pm.
Better from: Being carried, warmth (except teeth which are better from holding cold water in the mouth).

Cina

Worm Seed

The picture – mentals and generals

Cina produces symptoms commonly associated with worm infections and other abdominal irritations. Herbalists call it worm seed. Physically and mentally nervous. There is a constant irritation in the nose, causing a desire to rub it, press it, pick at it. It is a great children's remedy. Cross, badtempered, irritable, fretful children. Demanding and difficult to please. They have a tendency to stiffen out the body when cross or during cough. Capriciousness – desire for many things which they reject when offered them. Averse to touch and caresses, cannot bear having their head touched or stroked. They want to be rocked and carried. Easily offended by the slightest jest or teasing. Touchy. Nervous. Cross. Dissatisfied. Ravenous hunger. Restless sleep. Twitchings during the sleep. Grind the teeth during sleep. A remedy of night terrors. Child awakes from sleep in fright and cries out. Sour smelling children. Symptoms come on from anger, from excitement and from reprimands. Cough from anger. Convulsions in children after being reprimanded. Tossing about during sleep. Wetting of the bed. Ailments from anger and excitement.

Particular spheres of usefulness

Head: Ache, worse for reading or staring. Cannot bear having head touched or hair brushed.

Nose: Tremendous irritation; rubs and picks at nose till it bleeds.

Face: Pale with dark circles around eyes: bluish white around mouth; twitching of facial muscles and around eyes. One cheek red, the other pale.

Mouth: Grinds teeth during sleep; chewing motion during sleep.

Throat: Mucus in back of throat causing hawking.

Cough: Violent coughing attacks from a tickling sensation in throat, as of a feather; hawking from irritation of mucus. Cough excited by deep inspiration. Cough ending in spasm. Whooping cough. Child is afraid to move for fear of bringing on the cough. Gurgling noise from throat down to stomach after paroxysm of coughing.

Stomach: Voracious appetite; hunger soon after eating, or loss of appetite. Vomiting and diarrhoea immediately after eating and drinking. Aversion of baby to its mother's milk. Cravings for sweets and many different things.

Abdomen: Cutting, pinching pains from worms. Painful twisting about navel, better for pressure. Abdomen bloated, distended, hard and sore. Itching of anus. Loose white mucusy stool.

Urinary: Bedwetting. Urine turns milky on standing.

Extremities: Twitchings and jerkings. Stiffening out of whole body from vexation.

Sleep: Sleeplessness, particularly in children, with agitation and tearfulness; night terrors; rouses from sleep in fright and cries out: sleeps on abdomen or gets on hands and knees during sleep.

Fever: Fever with clean tongue; cold face and warm hands; much hunger.

Modalities: *Worse from*: Touch, worms, vexation, being looked at, during sleep, full moon, in sun, summer.
Better from: Lying on abdomen, motion, rocking.

Dulcamara

Bitter Sweet

The picture – mentals and generals

Dulcamara is particularly indicated in complaints coming on after, or aggravated by, exposure to wet, cold, damp weather or becoming suddenly chilled when heated; whether the symptoms be catarrhal, rheumatic, skin affections or whatever. Often required in the autumn, when warm days are followed by cold nights. Nose stuffs up when there is a cold rain. Catarrhal states, rheumatism, cough, stiff neck, eye troubles, earache, digestive troubles, skin troubles, urinary complaints and many others caused by the characteristics of Dulcamara – cold, wet, damp weather or becoming chilled when heated. Suppression of sweat from sudden chilling. Colds settle in the eyes or throat or affect the bladder, bowels or respiration. Many skin symptoms, eruptions, itching urticaria. Eruptions around the time of the menses; eruptions on the breast in nursing women; crusty, moist itching, bleeding eruptions. Rashes on babies. Eczema. Headaches from nasal catarrh becoming stopped. Pains around the navel gripping and pinching. Confusion of the mind, cannot concentrate thoughts. The Dulcamara patient wants to be warm; the catarrhal state is relieved by warm rooms, warm coverings. Tendency to warts. Can be irritable and impatient. Sometimes capricious.

Particular spheres of usefulness

Colds: Nose stuffs up in cold rain. Wants the nose warm. Coryza in newborn babies. Coryza fluent in warmth; stopped in cold air. Sneezing in cold air. Watery discharge from nose and eyes in open air. With the cold, eyes become sore and red, stiff neck, sore throat.

Cough: Cough provoked by tickling in throat with easy, loose expectoration.

Mouth: Increased flow of saliva, dry tongue. Thirst for cold drinks.

Abdomen: Colic and diarrhoea in cold, wet weather. Cutting, pinching pains around navel.

Urinary: Bladder inflammation coming on from characteristic causes – warm to cold and cold wet weather. Constant desire to urinate. Retention of urine from cold or from cold drinks.

Female: Rashes and eruptions around time of menses, itching eruptions on breasts in nursing women.

Neck: Stiff neck from cold.

Extremities: Rheumatic symptoms. Warts.

Skin: Urticaria: thick, moist, crusty, itching, bleeding eruptions. Rashes in newborns.

Modalities: *Worse from*: Becoming chilled when hot; cold, wet, damp weather; cold drinks, ice-creams; damp ground, damp rooms; autumn; getting feet wet or cold; suppressed discharges.
Better from: Moving about; warmth; dry weather.

Gelsemium

Yellow Jasmine

The picture – mentals and generals

Gelsemium is dull, drowsy, dizzy and droopy. Dazed and drooping. Dimness of vision or blurred vision preceding headache. Heaviness. Heavy head. Heavy, droopy eyes. Symptoms come on slowly over a period of several hours or several days. Gradually increasing lethargy and lassitude. Limbs feel heavy and weary, eyelids droop and feel too heavy to hold up. The skin takes on a dull, dusky pink flush and feels warm and moist to the touch. Trembling, particularly on attempting to move. Dizziness on attempting to move. Shivers and chills up and down the spine. Heavy head with congestive headache. Bursting headache extending to the forehead and eyes. Gelsemium complaints often come on in mild winters, in warm, wet weather. Summer influenzas and colds. Often useful after a bout of influenza when the patient cannot shake off the symptoms fully. They are not thirsty particularly. Do not want anything, except to be left alone in peace, to lie in bed, propped up on pillows so as to have the head held high. They have bouts of becoming active and excitable but soon become dizzy and weary and have to lie down again. Mentally and physically tired. Confusion of mind. Cannot think straight. Mild temperament. Gelsemium is often indicated in ailments from anticipation. Anticipatory anxiety and fears, fears of an ordeal, exams, interviews, dental treatment, travels by air and sea, stage fright, etc. Nervous anticipation which causes diarrhoea and trembling. Ailments from excitement. Fear of dark, falling, downward motion.

Particular spheres of usefulness

Head: Dull, heavy headache. Tight band sensation just above eyes and ears. Headache extending to neck and shoulders. Dizziness. Headache with blurred vision. Headache relieved by profuse urination.

Headache extending to forehead and eyeballs with bursting sensation. Congestive headache. Glazed, heavy eyes with big pupils, dusky, red face.

Eyes: Heavy, dull, drooping, blurred or dim sight preceding headaches.

Nose: Sneezing with fullness at root of nose. Congestion. Watery, excoriating discharge. Coryza like hot water in nostrils.

Face: Dull, dusky, flushed, pink, warm, moist skin. Droopy, dull expression.

Mouth: Tongue coated yellow.

Throat: Swallowing difficult, causes shooting pain into ear. Drinks regurgitate through the nose.

Colds: Symptoms come on slowly. Chills and shiverings up and down the back. Headache, congestive, with heaviness. Tickly cough. Coryza like hot water in the nostrils.

Influenza: Cold and fevers in mild, warm, wet, humid weather. Chills and shivering sensations up and down the spine, Bursting, congestive headaches with blurred vision, and heaviness, better from profuse urination, aching limbs with heaviness. Dizziness on attempting to move, also trembling.

Abdomen: Diarrhoea from nervous anticipation, frights and sudden emotions.

Urinary: Profuse urination ameliorates the headache. Involuntary urination in nervous children, from sudden surprises and frights.

Back/neck: Muscles feel aching and bruised. Relaxation of muscles. Sensation of chills and shivers up and down the spine.

Extremities: Deep, dull aching of all muscles. Trembling weariness, weakness and heaviness.

Fever: Chilliness, fatigue and aching in back and limbs with shivery sensations running up and down the back. The symptoms come on slowly with increasing weariness. Coming on in mild, warm, wet, humid weather or from becoming chilled when overheated. Wants to be held to stop him shaking so much.

Modalities: *Worse from*: Sudden emotions, excitement, dread, anticipation, warm humid weather, spring, summer, thunderstorms, foggy weather, motion.
Better from: Profuse urination, sweating, alcoholic drinks, lying down with head held high.

Hepar sulph.

Hepar Sulphuris Calcareum

The picture – mentals and generals

Hepar sulph. is extremely touchy, oversensitive, irritated and distraught by the slightest provocation – a word, a touch, the slightest pain, a draught of air. A very chilly patient worse in cold, damp weather. Extremely sensitive to cold, takes cold easily. Often indicated in respiratory and skin affections. Easy and profuse sweating without relief. Tendency to swollen glands. Tendency to suppuration. Offensive discharges which characteristically smell of cheese. Affects the skin and every little injury festers. Abscesses with sharp prickling pains or throbbing, exquisitively sensitive to touch and cold, can faint from the pain. Splinter sensations, sticking and pricking, sensation as of a fish bone in the throat. Quarrelsome. Abusive. Violent impulses. Sad and dejected. Dissatisfied. Hasty speech and hasty drinking. Cravings for vinegar and pickles, and condiments. Feels better from eating a meal. Years ago Hepar sulph. was famous as one of the effective croup remedies, the others being Aconite and Spongia, the indications for Hepar being a suffocative cough provoked by tightness of breath, rattling, anxious breathing, sense of suffocation with it. Cough aggravated by breathing in cold air, cough from any part of the body becoming uncovered, even a hand out of the bed clothes aggravates. Hepar is worse lying on the painful part. The side lain on becomes gradually very painful and he must turn over. Night sweats.

Particular spheres of usefulness

Ears: Discharges which are sometimes bad smelling. Increased wax.

Colds: Colds from exposure to cold air, cold wind – much catarrh. Better in moist, warm weather. Sneezing, stuffing up, discharge. Catarrh, smelling like old cheese. Sweats all night without relief. Easily chilled. Worse for draughts and inspiring cold air.

Cough: Cough worse from cold dry air, worse breathing in cold air, worse from any part of the body being uncovered, better in moist, warm weather. Hoarseness. Cough barking, suffocating, hacking. Rattling of mucus on chest. Expectoration loose, yellow and thick, becomes tight from cold air. Worse in dry, cold air, better in dry, clear weather or damp, warm weather.

Mouth: White pustules on inside of lips, cheek and tongue. Abscesses at roots of filled teeth. Unhealthy gums which ulcerate and bleed readily.

Face: Crack in middle of lower lip, pain in facial bones, worse touch. Eruptions in corner of lips.

Throat: Sensation as of a fish bone or splinter in throat on swallowing, extending to the ear on yawning. Pain on swallowing solids with rawness and scraping. Stitches extending to ear on swallowing.

Stomach: Craves acids, vinegar, wine, stimulants, strongly flavoured foods. Aversion to or craves fats. Acid risings.

Abdomen: Stitching in the right side, worse walking, touch, coughing, breathing. Diarrhoea after drinking cold water. Even soft stool is expelled with difficulty.

Urinary: Sensation that some urine remained in bladder after urinating. They must wait to urinate, then it passes slowly and without force.

Female: Leucorrhoea offensive, smelling like old cheese. Profuse perspiration during menopause.

Skin: Unhealthy – every little injury suppurates. Eruptions, particularly in the folds of skin. Abscesses, boils, carbuncles. Deep cracks on hands and feet.

Urticaria. Poor healing. Ulcers surrounded by little pimples. Cheesy discharges. All skin troubles are extremely sensitive to touch, to a breath of air. Easy and profuse sweat, sour and offensive.

Modalities: *Worse from:* Cold dry air. Cold winds, draughts, being uncovered. Any part becoming cold. Touch. Lying on painful part. Night, noise. Exertion.
Better from: Heat. Warm wraps, moist heat. Damp weather. After eating (comfortable feeling after eating is characteristic).

Ignatia

St Ignatius Bean

The picture – mentals and generals

Ignatia is a remedy which is full of surprises – contradictory, paradoxical states. Unexpected symptoms and modalities – sore throat which is better from swallowing rough foods; upset stomach which is better from hard to digest foods such as cabbages and onions; swollen, red joints which are not worse from touch and may even be better from it. Ignatia is overemotional, oversensitive and subject to rapidly changing moods. Hysterical tendencies, especially when they come on after a strain on the emotions. Suppressed emotions with inward brooding. Ailments from overstudying, overworking, worry, grief, disappointed love. They tend to fall in love with unsuitable people and enjoy being sad. Constant sighing and violent yawning. Overexcitable, trembling states with a tendency to faint easily. Nervous, sensitive and fearful. Fear of robbers. They are contrary. They cannot bear contradiction. Ignatia is a very chilly remedy. Cannot bear tobacco smoke. They are worse from drinking coffee. They feel much better from a change of position.

Particular spheres of usefulness

Head: Pain better from pressure. Headache from coffee, tobacco smoke, strong odours, sunlight, moving eyes, overstudying.

Eyes: Spasms of lids; flickering zigzags before the eyes. Watery eyes in bright sunlight.

Face: Alternate redness and paleness; one cheek hot and red; red face with chill.

Mouth: Toothache worse from coffee and smoking. Tendency to bite inside of cheeks whilst chewing or talking.

Throat: Sore throat. Stitching, shooting pains extending to ears, worse when not swallowing solids. Sensation of a lump in the throat which is better from eating solids. Globus hystericus.

Chest: Takes a deep breath for relief. Choking sensations. Coughing increases the desire to cough.

Stomach: Empty, sinking sensation in stomach, not better from eating, better from taking a deep breath. Desires acid things, fruit, cold things. Aversion to meat, milk, cooked foods, alcohol, tobacco. Hiccups coming on after eating, drinking or smoking.

Abdomen: Colicky, griping pain in one or both sides of abdomen. Abdominal pains are worse from coffee, brandy or things sweetened with sugar. Pain shoots upwards in rectum.

Heart: Palpitations worse at night. Anxious feeling with sinking, empty sensation in stomach.

Neck: Stiffness.

Sleep: Jerking of limbs on falling asleep. Violent yawning with watery eyes. Restless sleep. Disturbing dreams.

Fever: Red face and thirst during chill. Chill not relieved by external heat. Heat, without thirst, with aversion to uncovering. During fever violent itching, nettle rash over whole body. External heat with internal coldness.

Modalities: *Worse from*: Emotions. Grief, disappointment in love. Overtaxing the nervous system. Cold air. Touch. Coffee, tobacco. Stooping, walking, standing.

Better from: Change of position. Pressure to affected part. Taking a deep breath. Swallowing. Warmth. Sour things.

Lycopodium

Club Moss

The picture – mentals and generals

Lycopodium is a chilly patient, yet craves cool air, is worse in a warm, stuffy room. Desires sweet things and hot drinks. Snuffly babies. Children who are constantly hawking. An intellectual who is fearful of failure. Fears failure and does not attempt. In respiratory affections the nostrils are flared and flapping whilst the brow is wrinkled. The symptoms are generally worse from 4pm until 8pm. Wakes cross and irritable. Many stomach and abdominal symptoms. Easily full, even after eating only a small amount. Much dyspepsia with bloating, flatulence and belching. Feels full to bursting. Must loosen the clothing. Cannot stand tight belts. Oversensitive. A very fearful remedy – fear of the dark, fear of being alone, great fear in crowds, fear of ghosts. Anticipatory fears before undertaking any ordeal. Can be very restless. Many urinary symptoms – tormenting frequency with urging but must wait a long time before the urine will pass. Symptoms generally worse on the right side, travelling from right to left.

Particular spheres of usefulness

Head: Brow wrinkled, furrowed, particularly in respiratory affections; headaches worse in a warm room and worse lying down, better from cold air and from motion. Sick headache from going without a meal. Vertigo. Throbbing headache after coughing. Catarrhal headaches.

Colds: Nose stopped up. Snuffles, particularly of babies.

Sore throat generally worse on right side, worse from cold drinks and better for hot drinks. Sensation as if a ball is stuck in the throat. Food and drinks regurgitate through the nose. Nose stuffs up, worse at night, must breathe through the mouth. Fevers worse from 4–8pm.

Cough/ respiration: Dry, teasing, tickling cough; not much expectoration. Flapping of nostrils, forehead wrinkled with pain. Fevers rise 4–8pm. Short, rapid, rattling breathing. Tightness and burning in chest. Craves cold fresh air.

Stomach: Fullness after eating very little. Fullness, flatulence, bloating. Sensitive to pressure – cannot stand tight clothing. Craves sweets and hot drinks. Worse from cold food, flatulent, heavy foods. Worse from beans, cabbage, onions. Always belching.

Abdomen: Distension. Noisy flatulence. Better from empty eructations.

Urinary: Urging to urinate but must wait a long time before urine passes; feeling of heaviness in bladder; large quantities of urine passed during the night, quantity normal during the day. Pain before urinating.

Modalities: *Worse from*: 4–8pm. Pressure of clothes. Warmth. Eating to fullness. Oysters. Flatulent foods – beans, pastry, onion. Pressure.

Better from: Warm drinks. Warm food. Motion. Cool air. Eructations. Cold applications.

Nux vomica

Poison Nut

The picture – mentals and generals

Nux vomica is a remedy particularly suitable for the conditions which arise as a result of the modern way of life – fast pace, sedentary, overstimulated, high living. Nux symptoms often arise as a result of living under a good many mental strains, with irritability and late hours. Symptoms can come on suddenly. Overstimulated by coffee, rich foods, alcohol, tobacco and drugs of various kinds. The Nux patient stays up late at night, unable to sleep, a head full of thoughts and ideas and worries, only to wake late the next morning feeling hung-over. Particularly suited to morning after feelings – dull, headachey, liverish and tired. Nux vomica people are impatient, zealous, irascible, anxious to put all matters to rights and inclined to do it in a forceful and vehement way. It is said that he will tear off a button in fury if it does not go his way whilst dressing. Nux is highly sensitive to injustice. Unafraid of conflict they often speak their minds. Spasms and cramps and easily faint. Constipation – ineffectual urging, incomplete stool. Many stomach symptoms. Patient feels he would be better if he could be sick, but cannot. A very chilly patient. During fever cannot uncover in the least, even a hand, without feeling chilly. An overstrained nervous system, hypersensitive, irritable, passionate in his belief and volatile in his methods of putting things to rights. Persons who have taken many drugs. Very sensitive to strong odours. The consequences of disappointed ambitions and injured pride. Nervous debility from excesses. Violent impulses. Demanding. Wants to have things his own way. Craves something to brace him up. Generally worse early morning. Faints from odours. Faints from every labour pain. Cannot tolerate the least smell, noise or movement. Very sensitive to music, weeping from music. Easily offended. Restless.

Particular spheres of usefulness

Head: Aches after indulgence in late hours, rich foods, alcohol and stimulants. Worse early morning. Faintness. Dizziness. Intoxicated feeling with confusion. Frontal headache with desire to press head against something. Headache with constipation and piles. Heaviness and sensation of expansion as if forehead would burst. Sore, oversensitive scalp. Worse for stimulants and mental exertion.

Colds: Stuffy colds, especially coming on in cold, dry weather. Oversensitive to odours – may faint from odours. Fluent coryza in daytime – stopped nose at night. Snuffles of newborn babies. Fluent in open air – stopped up in a warm room. Violent sneezing. Colds with headaches and chilliness. Unbearable itching of nostrils.

Ears: Itching in ears and through eustachian tube, which compels swallowing.

Mouth: Toothache which is worse from cold things and better from warm drinks.

Abdomen: Ineffectual urging to stool. Irregular sore bowels, worse from coughing and jarring. Has to strain at stool, feels as if not all is expelled. Piles, bleeding, itching. Constipation. Unsatisfactory stools.

Stomach: Dyspepsia. Acidity with nausea. Wants to vomit for relief, but cannot. Desires coffee, tea, wine, stimulants, rich foods. Loves fats and tolerates them well. Heaviness and pain in stomach. Stomach sensitive to pressure.

Female: Fainting during menses. Cramping pains during menses with urging to stool. Labour pains unbearable, with fainting.

Extremities: Knee joint cracking during motion.

Fever: Whole body hot and face red and burning hot, yet cannot uncover **in the least** without feeling chilly. Must be covered in every stage of the fever.

Modalities: *Worse from*: Cold, dry weather. Early morning. Uncovering. Alcohol, drugs, stimulants. Slightest cause. Pressure of clothes.

Better from: Discharges. Naps, resting. Milk, fats, hot drinks. Covering head. Warm, wet weather.

Pulsatilla

Wind Flower

The picture – mentals and generals

Pulsatilla is often called the weathercock remedy on account of its wandering, changeable symptoms. Also mentally changeable.

Smiles and tears follow each other with great rapidity. Pulsatilla is suitable for people who are mild of temperament, shy, slow in movement, easily moved to tears, irresolute, easily influenced and easily discouraged. Two of the chief indications for Pulsatilla are: better from slow movement and better from cool, fresh, open air. Strong desire for cool air. General desire for cold things, air, food, drinks, applications, and they feel better for them. Even when chilly they feel much worse in a warm, stuffy room. Pulsatilla is very useful in complaints which come on after getting wet, particularly after getting the feet wet. Pulsatilla is touchy, and can be irritable, sensitive to every slight, even imagined ones. They are sympathetic and desire company, sympathy and affection. Clingy children who do not like to be left alone and are shy with strangers. Gentle, pitiful crying. Pulsatilla has a strong effect on the digestion and they are easily upset by rich fatty foods and pastries. Dryness of the mouth without thirst. Inclined to lie with the head high and the hands over the head. The typical Pulsatilla discharges are yellowish green, thick and bland. Symptoms always changing. Fearful of the dark and of being left alone. Jealous and suspicious. Self-pitying and dependent.

Particular spheres of usefulness

Head: Aches with menstrual or digestive symptoms or from overwork. Better from cold, from pressure and sometimes from slow motion.

Eyes: Burning, itching causing patient to rub them. Inflamed lids. Styes, thick, yellow, bland discharges.

Ears: Thick yellow discharges. Ear troubles following colds and eruptive dis-eases. Hearing difficult, as if ears stopped up.

Mouth: Dryness without thirst. Toothache better from cold.

Nose: Catarrhal conditions with loss of smell and taste. Thick, bland, yellow discharges. Watery discharges and sneezing. Stuffing up in a warm room and at night and lying down, better from being out in open air. Nosebleed from suppressed menses.

Cough: Cough worse in a warm room, in the evening when lying down. Dry at night, loose during the day. Gagging and choking. Wants cold air. Must sit up in bed. Cough after measles.

Stomach: Disordered stomach from indulgence in rich foods, pastries, pork, ice-creams, onions. Not thirsty. Desires sour and refreshing things. Aversion to fats and pork. Bad taste in mouth. Flatulence after eating.

Abdomen: Pressure as of a stone. Painful, distended, loud rumbling. Slow digestion.

Female: Menses late, scanty, changeable. Delayed from getting feet wet. Weak, irregular, flitting labour pains. Breech position of baby.

Respiratory: Short breath, worse lying on left side. Smothering sensation on lying down. Worse if heated, better from open air and sitting up.

Extremities: Drawing, tearing pains in limbs, wandering from place to place. Inclination to stretch the limbs. Painful red swollen joints. Veins full and swollen. Legs feel heavy and weary. Complaints worse when limbs hanging down.

Skin: Itching worse in evening, worse for warmth. Sensitive to wool. Rashes like measles. Swollen glands. Eruptions after pork and rich foods. Varicose veins, moles.

Sleep: Sleeps with hands over head, head high.

Fever: Chilliness without thirst, averse to heat. One-sided perspiration, partial heat, partial chilliness. Heat with distended veins.

Modalities: *Worse from*: Warmth. Rich fatty foods. Getting wet. Letting limbs hang down. Puberty. Evening (mental symptoms). Morning (digestive symptoms). Lying on left side.

Better from: Cold fresh air. Slow gentle motion. Lying with head high. Pressure, rubbing.

Rhus toxicodendron

Poison Ivy

The picture – mentals and generals

Rhus tox. is most often indicated by its causation and aggravation. Causation – exposure to cold, damp, wet weather, sitting on damp ground, cold bathing, drinking cold water, particularly when heated. Rhus tox. has a very marked aggravation on first beginning to move after a period of rest – pain and stiffness on first movement which eases after moving around a while. The Rhus tox. patient is better from continued movement. Very restless – must be continually changing position to get relief. In fever the patient will be very restless, continually changing position and tossing about the bed. Anxiety, fear, irritability restlessness. Weakness from continuing moving but compelled to move to ease the pains. Craving for cold drinks but they bring on the chills. Craves cold milk. Often indicated in rheumaticky aches, pains and stiffness, muscular aches, drawing, tearing pains in and around joints, sore, bruised sensation, lameness. Rhus tox. is relieved by continual motion, heat and rubbing. Often indicated following sprains and strains, for which it is very useful as a first aid measure. Soreness of muscles and tendons from overlifting. Complains after any over-exertion. Eruptions and blisters which burn and itch. Anxiety, weeping without knowing why.

Particular spheres of usefulness

Face:	Neuralgia with chilliness. Lips dry, cracked, with eruptions.
Mouth:	Tongue dry, cracked, has a triangular red tip.
Colds and influenza:	From wet weather, cold, damp. Throat red, swollen, puffy. Hoarseness, rawness, roughness – worse on first beginning to sing or talk, better after

talking or singing a little while. Thirst for cold drinks, but they bring on the chills and cough. Worse for uncovering, even a hand. Much sneezing and coughing. Aching in bones of the nose. Bones aching. Thick yellow mucus, offensive smell. Weakness. Restlessness. Hot, dry skin.

Cough/ respiration: Dry, teasing cough. Worse at night. Hoarseness from overstraining the voice. Rust coloured expectoration. Pain and difficult breathing worse from rest. Must move about. Restless.

Stomach: Craves cold drinks but they bring on the chills and cough. Very thirsty. Desires cold milk.

Abdomen: Diarrhoea. Piles. Worse lifting, straining. Colic. Better for motion.

Neck/back: Stiff neck. Backache, better for pressure, movement. Stiffness. Bruised sensation, worse resting.

Extremities: Sprains and strains. Pains, rheumaticky, coming on after exposure to cold damp air and after overexertion. Stiffness, numbness, tingling, puffiness, lameness. Soreness, bruised sensation. Soreness from overlifting. Drawing pains in and around joints. Joints hot, painful, swollen. Worse wet. Better warm, dry applications. Worse first movement. Better continued movement. Red, shiny, smooth swellings.

Skin: Eruptions, blisters, rashes. Intense itching, burning, tingling. Must scratch which increases the desire to scratch.

Fever: Slow fevers. Very thirsty for cold drinks, which bring on chills and cough. Very restless. Continually moving about for relief. Tongue coated, dry, cracked, hot. Aching in bones. Chills worse for uncovering – even a hand. Worse at night. Aching in back. Dry skin. Very weak. Prostrated, but compelled to keep moving. From cold damp weather, particularly when perspiring. Worse in winter and before a storm. Better from change of position.

Modalities: *Worse from*: Wet, cold, damp. Chilled when perspiring. Uncovering. First beginning to move after

a rest. Rest. Before storms. Sprains and strains. Over-exertion. Cold drinks.
Better from: Continued motion. Heat – hot bath, warm wraps. Warm dry applications. Rubbing. Change of position. Stretching limbs. Warm dry weather. Holding affected part.

Spongia

Roasted Sponge

The picture – mentals and generals

Spongia has great dryness of the air passages. Often indicated in coughs, particularly croupy types of cough. Dry coryza. Stuffed nose. Cough is dry, barking, crowing, wheezy, whistling, hollow, tight; often sounds like a saw driven through a board. Seldom is there any rattling of mucus with Spongia – everything is tight and dry. Dry asthma. Cough coming on from exposure to cold dry air, cold dry winds. Symptoms usually coming on slowly over the course of a day or two. Hoarseness, soreness and rawness; dryness and burning. Larynx very sensitive to touch and voice becoming weak or hoarse from singing or talking. Aggravation on lying down. Rousing from sleep with a suffocative sensation; with alarm and anxiety; difficult breathing. Worse from lying with the head low. Better from warm food and drink. Worse at night. Worse from cold drinks.

Particular spheres of usefulness

Cough/ respiratory: Dryness of air passages. Coughs, colds, croup. Hoarseness; voice gives out when singing or talking. Rawness and soreness and burning. Sensitive to touch and noise. Dry asthma. Symptoms coming on after exposure to cold dry winds. Cough is croupy, hollow, barking, wheezy. Seldom is there any rattling of mucus. Worse at night and worse lying with head low. Rouses from sleep in fright and alarm with suffocative sensation; difficult breathing. Feels choking on lying down to go to sleep. Worse from cold drinks, sweets, excitement. Sore throat worse from sweets. Better from eating a little warm food and better sometimes from warm drinks. Constantly clearing throat.

Modalities: *Worse from*: Dry, cold, wind, after sleep, exertion, full moon, sweets.
Better from: Lying with head low, eating or drinking a little, warm things, descending.

Sulphur

Flowers of Sulphur, the Element

The picture – mentals and generals

Sulphur is one of the most widely used of all remedies. It can be very useful in acute conditions when the symptoms fit. It is often very useful in finishing acute infectious illnesses. Whilst the classic type who requires Sulphur is the stoop-shouldered, untidy philosopher it can be useful for anyone when the symptoms demand it. A hot, warm-blooded patient; the soles of the feet often become burning hot in bed so he thrusts them out of the covers. His skin is often apt to be itchy and aggravated by heat and woollen clothes. Generally starving at 11am; desire for sweet things and fatty foods. Dread of being washed. Burnings; itching eruptions. Redness particularly around the rims of the eyes, redness of nostrils, lips. Flushes of heat – often useful in women at the menopause. Babies who are always hungry and warm and sweaty, kick off their covers. Dry rough skin. Always tired; likes to have catnaps; worse standing. Empty, weak and faint at 11am or an hour before a meal is due. Sulphur can also prefer to drink rather than eat. Generally lazy. Mentally full of ideas but too lazy to do anything about them. An armchair philosopher. Self-centred. Critical. Effects of alcohol. Worse from too much heat or too much cold. Restless. Wishing to touch something. Illusions that anything he takes a fancy to is beautiful – old rags, old sticks. Full of pride. Daydreams. Argumentative, irritable, impatient. Enthusiastic, easily excited, oversensitive.

Particular spheres of usefulness

Head:	Headaches from going without a meal. Headaches from indulgence in alcohol. Burning sensation on top of head; much itching which turns to a burning sensation on being scratched. Hot head, cold feet. Sick headaches with nausea and vomiting. Aches worse when stooping. Vertigo worse when standing, stooping.
Eyes:	Heat, burning and itching of eyes and lids; pain in eyes, extending to head, worse in sunlight, worse for movement; sensitive to light. Redness of rims and eyelids.
Ears:	Very red; burning heat; itchings.
Face:	Lips dry, rough, very red; heat of cheeks, redness, burning sensations.
Nose:	Itching, burning and redness of nostrils; offensive odour before nose.
Throat:	Burning redness and dryness. Sore throat. Swollen tonsils. Sensation as of a hard ball rising in throat.
Colds:	Nose stopped. Discharges from nose acrid, burning, watery. Sneezing. Colds coming on from cold air, becoming overheated, taking a bath. Fluent discharge alternating with stoppage of nose. Sensitive to draughts and cold open air; worse from bathing and washing.
Cough/ respiration:	Oppressed respiration, wants windows open for fresh air; sensation of heat in chest – or of coldness; pains in chest extending to back – worse for coughing, deep breathing, lying on back. Congestions. Burning sensations.
Stomach:	Craves sweet things; craving for fat; always hungry; or drinks much, eats little, fainting, weak, empty at 11am or an hour before meal is due. Milk

aggravates; desires apples and raw foods; nausea during pregnancy; acidity, sour eructations.

Abdomen: Sensation of soreness; sensitive to pressure; colic after food or fullness, heaviness, pressure. Early morning diarrhoea driving him out of bed. Redness, itching and burning of anus; piles itching, burning. Constipation – stool large, hard, dry, difficult, painful. Stool unsatisfactory – not completely expelled.

Urinary: Constant desire to urinate – a few drops pass involuntarily, must hurry. Frequent urination particularly at night; bedwetting particularly in warm children who love sugar, love fats, hate being washed.

Skin: Eruptions of every kind, itching, burning like fire, must scratch till it bleeds, worse from night, heat, washing. Sensitive to woollens and synthetic clothing. Skin red, rough, dry, cracked; looks dirty even after washing. Skin burns when scratched.

Fever: Flushes of heat throughout body; perspiration of single parts; night sweats. External heat with internal chilliness and a red face. Sleeps in catnaps. Sleepy during day, wakeful at night. Talks and twitches during sleep. Throws off the covers. Soles of feet burn and he puts them out into the cool air. Prevented from falling asleep by flow of thoughts.

Modalities: *Worse from:* Warmth, warmth of bed, washing, 11am, standing, stooping, milk, suppressions, overexertion, sweets, reaching high.

Better from: Warm, dry weather (not too hot or too cold), drawing up affected limbs, motion, lying on right side.

Part Four

10. The First Aid Remedies

First aid remedies and their uses

The first aid remedies are the easiest remedies to use because they are prescribed for specific injuries, rather than conditions which arise from within. Unlike the general remedies previously described, you do not need to individualize the patient to prescribe them. Use the first aid remedies required according to the directions described under each of them. Use of the first aid remedies is the closest that homoeopathy comes to herbalism. All of these remedies come from the plant world. Whilst Arnica, Rhus tox. and some of the first aid remedies do have a use in individualized homoeopathy, their main use in the home will be found in the first aid situation.

At-a-glance guide to the first aid remedies' spheres of usefulness

Arnica Physical trauma of any kind, bumps, bruises, sprains, strains, aching, sore muscles (see page 101)
Calendula After dentition, mouth ulcers, bites, stings, spots, cuts (see pages 101–2)
Ledum Bites, stings, punctured wounds, severe bruising, blood blisters, black eyes (see page 103)
Hypericum Deep wounds, crushed or stubbed fingers and toes (see page 103)
Symphytum Bruising to bones, shins, cheek, forearm, etc., fractures, broken bones, eye injuries (see page 104)
Urtica urens Burns (see page 104)
Ruta Bruises, strained or torn ligaments and tendons (see page 105)
Rhus tox. Strains, sprains (see page 105)

Bellis perennis Bruising to soft tissue, after operations (injury to internal soft tissue), old injuries (see pages 106–107)

Arnica montana

Arnica should definitely be in everyone's home medicine chest. It is the chief accident remedy. It is also known as Leopards Bane and Fall Herb. It is a member of the daisy family and has a beautiful orangey-yellow daisylike flower. It grows on mountain sides in Europe, ready to help those who have fallen and suffered injury. Local people make it into a tea to use in cases of accidents and many collect it during the summer to dry in readiness for the winter months.

It is the first remedy to be given following a physical trauma of any kind – bumps, bruises, sprains and strains; also for tired, sore, aching muscles due to overexertion. The key symptom is *soreness*. It should be given before and following dental treatment, operations, childbirth, as it relieves the pain, assists in recovery from shock and aids recovery. It can even be useful after a long aeroplane journey where the person feels thrown about and bruised inside. It can even be given in concussion by dissolving the pillule in a small amount of water and moistening the tongue with it at frequent intervals.

In all cases it should be given in potency 30 or 6 every two or three hours, or more frequently in more severe cases, for three or four doses, or until relief is obtained.

It can be applied externally to unbroken skin – twelve drops of the tincture to one tablespoon of cold water as a compress, especially in sprains and strains and bruises, but *it must not be applied to broken surfaces* as it may cause irritation.

Calendula

This is the English Marigold, another member of the daisy family with lovely orangey-yellow petals. It is most often used externally to promote healing of injured skin, for cuts, burns and stings. It stimulates the formation of new healthy tissue and prevents sepsis. Although it is not an antiseptic in the strict sense of the word, in that it does not actually kill bacteria, it does inhibit the growth of micro-organisms, so that they do not thrive in its presence. It is used for treating all cuts, wounds, sore places and bruises where the skin is broken. If a wet dressing is needed, dilute the tincture 1:25 with water and apply a piece of lint soaked in the solution, covered with a piece of cotton wool and bandaged. When it gets dry the lint should be damped without removing. It is important to keep it damp.

This solution, Calendula 1:25 with water, is also very useful as a mouthwash after the removal of teeth, or when there are mouth ulcers.

It is useful in bites, stings, septic spots and also burns (after Urtica Urens has commenced the healing process). It stimulates the healthy growth of new cells. It is also useful after childbirth – the dilution applied to the perineum will soothe and aid healing if torn or cut.

Calendula is best used in superficial wounds as, if the wound is deep, Calendula will heal it and seal it too quickly before dirt has had a chance to come out. In such cases, Hypericum is better.

In an emergency the fresh flowers, crushed first to release their essential properties, can be applied to a wound or sting.

Calendula was used a lot in the American Civil War and the First World War, with many accounts of praise to the staff of wards in which it was used for the lack of incidence of sepsis and the quick recovery of the patients therein. It stops bleeding and does this quicker if applied undiluted, although it does sting at first so is best diluted. The bleeding usually gets temporarily worse and then just stops. It is useful as a mouthwash after tooth extraction to stop the bleeding. It is well worthwhile to grow some Marigold flowers in your garden. The wild variety is better than the cultivated, so if allowed to seed and the seed replanted they will, after a few seasons, revert to a more natural and healthy variety. It can also be bought as a cream which is very soothing for dry, cracked, sore skin and lips.

Ledum palustre

Ledum, or the Marsh Tea, is especially useful for punctured wounds made by sharp instruments, such as rusty nails; also for animal bites and insect stings; also splinters under the nail. It takes the pricking pain out of these wounds, especially where the patient prefers cold dressings to hot ones. It also prevents sepsis if given early enough. It is given as often as necessary according to the severity of the injury – generally repeat the dose whenever the pain returns. It is used in potency 6c.

Another use of Ledum is in cases of severe bruising, black eyes, blood blisters, where there is great extravasation of blood. Arnica should be given first for bruising but if the Arnica is not enough to take it away, then Ledum will follow on well, absorb the blood and so reduce the swelling and bruising. The affected part feels cold, yet is relieved by cold applications.

Hypericum

Hypericum perforatum is the wild St John's Wort, which grows in hedgerows and fields. Hypericum is especially indicated when parts rich in nerves are injured, as in crushed or stubbed toes and fingers. There is excessive painfulness, the pains are shooting; they shoot along the course of a nerve. It is also indicated after falls on the coccyx. It is useful anywhere where nerves are affected. Useful after operations. It is also useful after animal bites or insect stings, where the pain shoots up the limb.

It is used internally, in potency 6c, several doses at intervals between fifteen minutes and four hours, depending on the severity of the pain. As in all cases the doses should be discontinued as soon as relief is obtained and only started again if the pain returns. It is also used externally in the form of a tincture or cream. The tincture is diluted 1:25 as the Calendula. It is best used for dressing wounds which are rather too deep for Calendula.

Symphytum

Symphytum, better known by the name Comfrey, used to be called Knitbone and Boneset. *Symphio-* is a Greek word meaning to unite, which indicates the special affinity it has with bones. It has a powerful action in cell proliferation and especially when concerned with bones. It is used specifically for bruised periosteum, the outer covering of the bone, which is particularly vulnerable where the bone comes near the surface, as in the shin bone and cheek bone, and for fractured and broken bones, to hasten healing and cause the parts to unite more quickly. It is also useful for eye injuries caused by a blunt instrument.

For fractured bones, first use Arnica for two or three days, second Ledum for two or three days, third Symphytum for seven to ten days to aid nature in the healing of the bony tissues. Use potency 6c in all cases.

Urtica urens

Urtica urens, otherwise known as the humble but excellent stinging nettle which causes such stinging, burning pains on contact with the skin, is also very efficacious in removing such pains when applied to a burned area, in tincture form. It can either be used neat or diluted 1:25 with water. It is very useful kept in the kitchen and gives instant relief when dabbed on fingers that have touched hot saucepans or even for a burned tongue from tasting something too hot. It does take away the pain from these burns and should be reapplied should the pain return.

For larger burns, cover burned areas with a wet cloth soaked in the diluted Urtica tincture (or a mixture of urtica and Calendula tincture). Also take the Urtica urens internally in potency 30c. This is, of course, in the case of painful but nevertheless minor burns, which one would treat at home anyway. In more severe cases medical help must be called but, meanwhile this remedy can be given while waiting.

Ruta graveolens

Ruta, or Rue, is the chief remedy for bruised and fractured bones, especially the periosteum, therefore it is very useful for bruises after kicks on the shin in footballers, etc. Bruised sensations, with restlessness. Also useful for strained and torn tendons and ligaments, sprained wrists and ankles. A very beneficial remedy to take away pain and inflammation from torn ligaments and synovial membranes around joints, especially the small joints.

In any of these injuries, give Arnica, the initial injury remedy, as usual, then follow it up with Ruta 6c every two hours, or more often depending on severity of pain, for two or three days, thereafter repeating if and when pain occurs. Ruta is also indicated for restoring the eyesight to normal when it has become dim from straining the muscles by too much close work – reading, writing and sewing, etc.

Rhus toxicodendron

Rhus tox., or the Poison Ivy, is very useful for strains and sprains from overexertion. The key symptom is worse on first movement, then better after some continued movement. In sprained wrists and ankles, think of Arnica and Rhus tox. In painful swelling of joints worse for rest and better from gentle movement, think of Rhus tox. Use potency 6c three hourly for up to five to six days. Continue as necessary.

Bellis perennis

The English daisy is very useful for internal shocks and bruising particularly. The effects of a blow to soft tissues. Useful for the effects of a sudden chill to an internal or external body surface, e.g. a cold drink on a hot day. Very useful for the after effects of operations, i.e. the injury and shock to internal tissues. Useful for effects of injuries, leaving a part weakened. It has been called the gardeners' remedy, being useful for all the sprains and strains they may suffer. In acute cases use potency 6c two hourly for three to four days. In old injuries take the 30th potency night and morning for three days.

11. Conclusion

If this book has value we hope that it is mainly to help you on your way to the unfolding of your ideals and dreams of freedom from dis-ease and fear. To practise homoeopathy one needs, as we hope has been made plain, to suspend judgement and prejudice. If you come away with the possibility of operating from an unprejudiced and holistic viewpoint then we will have achieved our aim. We do not believe that homoeopathy is, alone, the sole road to health and freedom from dis-ease. It is one of many roads that all lead to the same place, namely health of mind, body and spirit. Hahnemann himself operated from this holistic viewpoint. He saw his patients as more than blood and bones wrapped up in skin. He realized that mankind had a higher self that, if thwarted in its freedom of expression, would create disagreeable symptoms in order to make its unease known. The attributes which one must learn in order to use the laws of homoeopathy successfully will serve for many worthwhile uses and help in many endeavours. Lack of prejudice, a holistic view, a belief in health and freedom and a trust in eternal laws can only be beneficial to us as human beings. Those who have read these chapters will, we hope, not only have gained an insight into this truly rational art of healing but will also have realized the confidence and practical ability to apply its principles in a rational and appropriate way. Also, those wishing to take their studies further will have a firm foundation on which to build.

There is a growing band of people who are interested in learning more about homoeopathy for home use. The needs of these people are well served in the many homoeopathy groups which exist countrywide. Those wishing to extend their knowledge of remedies beyond the scope of this book may obtain advice and information from these types of groups. Homoeopaths are regularly invited to speak to members and meetings centre around lively and informal discussions on any aspect of homoeopathy. Also a growing number of adult education centres run evening courses on first aid and basic homoeopathy. Contact your local Citizens Advice Bureau or your library for more information.

If your prime interest is in receiving homoeopathic treatment from a professional, this guide may well serve to clear up some questions and anxieties that you may have. Those already using homoeopathy as part of their health care may find the indepth view this book offers provides a greater understanding of their own treatment.

Professional homoeopaths come from three backgrounds. There are the regular doctors who, having completed their training in allopathic medicine, can choose to study homoeopathy at the Faculty of Homoeopathy in London. On successful completion of the course they are awarded the Title MFHom. There are also a variety of colleges which specialize in teaching homoeopathy to a professional standard for lay practitioners. The first College of Homoeopathy was started by what was to become the Society of Homoeopaths in 1978. These are usually part-time courses running from three to four years. Information is available from the Institute of Complementary Medicine (see Useful Addresses). Last, but not least, are the homoeopaths who have learnt homoeopathy through the traditional method of apprenticeship and self-study.

To find a homoeopath suited to you, personal recommendation is often the best road. However, information on where to find a homoeopath who is registered with the Faculty or the Society can be obtained from the Institute of Complementary Medicine and the British Homoeopathic Association in London. Many useful addresses covering all aspects of homoeopathic interest have been provided at the back of the book. For those readers requiring information on homoeopathy in USA, Canada, Australia, New Zealand and South Africa, contact the relevant associations.

It is the authors' firm belief that the more people use homoeopathy, with a full, holistic understanding of what they are doing, the healthier and less susceptible to dis-ease will mankind be. Our health is our responsibility. Homoeopathy gives us the chance to accept the challenge to learn how to recognize, recover and preserve it. May your road be straight and your load light.

Wishing you well,

Nigel and Susan Garion-Hutchings.

Answers to Test Cases

Test case No.1	Remedy: Aconite.
Test case No.2	Remedy: Gelsemium.
Test case No.3	
Categories:	
Mode of onset:	Came on gradually
Possible cause:	Exposure to hot sun
Mental/emotional:	Irritability, impatience, worries about work
General:	Hot and dry, thirsty (for long cold drinks of water), dizzy and faint (on sitting up)
Particular:	Throat – sore, red, dry Headache – throbbing
Modalities	
Mental/emotional:	Irritability < answering questions
General:	> fresh air, > keeping still, < stuffy rooms
Particular:	headache < movement, < thinking, < stuffy rooms, > pressure, > keeping still
Remedy:	Bryonia

Glossary

Abstinence To go without.
Aconite Remedy made from Monkshead flower.
Acrid Bitter or irritating to taste or smell.
Aggravation Temporary intensification of symptoms.
Allopath Orthodox medical doctor.
Ameliorate To relieve symptoms.
Antidote Something that works against an unwanted condition.
Aperient A laxative, mildly cathartic.
Aphorism A concise statement of principle.
Apis mellifica Remedy made from the sting of the bee.
Arnica montana Remedy made from a mountain flower.
Arsenicum album Remedy made from Arsenic.
Assimilation Transformation of food to living tissue.
Belladonna Remedy made from Deadly Nightshade.
Bellis perennis Remedy made from the Daisy flower.
Bloodletting To drain blood from a person.
Calcarea carbonica Remedy made from Calcium carbonate.
Calendula Tincture or dilution made from the Marigold flower.
Carbo vegetabilis Remedy made from vegetable carbon.
Carbuncles Small growths found on the feet.
Catalyst Something which triggers another reaction.
Centesimal Divided into hundreds or based upon divisions into hundreds.
Chamomilla Remedy made from the Chamomile flower.
Characteristic symptoms Symptoms which are distinguishing features.
Cina Remedy made from 'Worm Seed'.
Coccyx Small 'tail' bone at bottom end of spine.
Common symptoms Symptoms found in every case.

Compress A pad of linen holding herbs or other treatments in place with pressure.
Convulsions Violent involuntary contractions of the muscles.
Coryza Acute catarrhal condition with nasal discharge.
Croup Resonant, barking cough found chiefly in children and infants.
Cystitis Inflammation of the bladder causing irritation and pain.
Dietetics The science of study and regulation of the diet.
Dilated Enlarged, widened beyond the normal dimensions.
Discharge A setting free or substance evacuated.
Dis-ease Lack of ease causing symptoms and distress.
Distended Enlarged.
Dulcamara Remedy made from the plant *Solanum dulcamara*.
Dynamic level The energy level.
Dynamic plane The energy plane.
Dynamization A method of energizing a medicine to increase its effectiveness.
Emotional sphere Pertaining to any emotional activity.
Equilibrium A balance.
Eructation A belch.
Eustachian tube A fine tube about 1½ inches long connecting the middle ear to the air passages.
Excoriating Causing irritation and soreness.
Expectoration Coughing up material from the lungs, bronchi and trachea: sputum.
Flatulent Having or producing gas in the stomach or intestines.
Fontanelles Membrane covered spaces found on top of a baby's skull.
Gagging Choking.
Gelsemium Remedy made from the root of *Gelsemium sempervirens*.
Hepar sulph. Remedy made from Calcium sulphide.
Holistic The whole picture, not just a part or parts.
Homoeopathic That which is harmonious to the whole.
Homoeopathy The medical practice of treating like with like in order to stimulate a cure.
Hypericum A remedy made from the plant *Hypericum perforatum*.

Hystericus Symptom brought on by over-excitement.
Ignatia Remedy made from the seeds of *Strychnos ignatia.*
Inert Not active.
Inspiration The act of inhaling.
Ledum palustre Remedy made from the fresh herb *Ledum palustre.*
Leucorrhoea Vaginal discharge.
Lycopodium A remedy made from the pollen of *Lycopodium clavatum.*
Malady Illness.
Metaphysical A consideration of the origin of things and the nature of being.
Materia Medica Manual containing remedy descriptions.
Menses Monthly periods.
Mental sphere Pertaining to all mental activity.
Modalities That which influences symptoms for the better or worse.
Morbific influence Any harmful influence.
Morbific stimulus That which stimulates harmful influences.
Neuralgia Severe pain along the course of a nerve.
Nux vomica A remedy made from the seeds of Strychnos Nux vomica.
Optimum health A maximum level of health.
Organon A work by Samuel Hahnemann describing his homoeopathic findings and his life's work.
Orthodox Conforming to the usual beliefs or established doctrines.
Palliative To lessen the severity without curing.
Palpitations Rapid heartbeat or fluctuations.
Paroxysm A sudden attack.
Pathology All the symptoms of a particular disease as viewed from an allo-pathic point of view.
Periosteum Live cellular covering of the bones.
Physical sphere Relating to all physical aspects of life.
Pillule Small pill.
Potency Strength of remedy.
Potentization Act of energizing and increasing safety and effectiveness of medicines through dilutions and succussions.
Prostration Laid low, overcome, physically weak and exhausted.

Provers Those that tried and tested substances to establish their homoeopathic values.
Provings Written accounts of provers' experiences.
Pulsatilla A remedy made from the Wind flower.
Purging A forceful cleansing.
Pustules Spots containing pus.
Retching The straining action of vomiting without bringing anything up.
Rhus toxicodendron A remedy made from the fresh leaves of the Poison Ivy.
Ruta graveolens A remedy made from the fresh plant *Ruta graveolens*.
Sensation A conscious feeling.
Septic Micro-organisms that are infecting or putrefying.
Sepsis A poisoning of the blood due to certain micro-organisms.
Similia similibus curantur Treating like with like.
Similimum The most similar remedy
Spasm Involuntary contraction of a muscle.
Spasmodic Fitful, intermittent.
Spongia A remedy made from Turkey sponge, toasted brown.
Succussion Process of dilution and shaking/ banging.
Sulphur A remedy made from Sulphur.
Suppurate To form or discharge pus.
Suppressant Anything which is used to force-fully prohibit or restrain.
Symphytum A remedy made from the Comfrey herb.
Symptomatology Any condition or circumstance that accompanies something and indicates its existence.
Symptom picture A collection of all symptoms of the case to give a 'whole picture'.
Tincture A substance in a solution of alcohol.
Ulceration An infected open sore.
Urticaria A skin rash.
Urtica urens A remedy made from the Stinging Nettle.
Uvula The small fleshy part of the soft palate hanging down above the back of the tongue.
Venesection Cutting into a vein.
Vertigo A sensation of dizziness.

Vital force The energizing principle that pervades all living things. The vital principle behind life. Sometimes known as the 'tao' or 'chi'.

\> Is better for:–

< Is worse for:–

Further Reading

Livingston, R. *Homoeopathy – Born 1810, Still Going Strong*, Asher Press, 1973.

Roberts, H. *The Principles and Art of Cure by Homoeopathy*, Health Science Press/C.W. Daniel, 1962.

Puddephatt, Noel, *Puddephatt's Primers*, C.W. Daniel, 1976.

Shepherd, D. *Homoeopathy for the First Aider*, Health Science Press/ C.W. Daniel, 1972.

Shepherd, D. *Homoeopathy in Epidemic Diseases*, Health Science Press/ C.W. Daniel, 1967.

Shepherd, D. *Magic of the Minimum Dose*, Health Science Press/C.W. Daniel, 1946.

Shepherd D. *More Magic of the Minimum Dose*, Health Science Press/ C.W. Daniel, 1974.

Speight, P. *Homoeopathy – A Practical Guide to Natural Medicine*, Grafton Books, 1979.

Tyler, M.L. *Homoeopathic Drug Pictures*, Health Science Press/ C.W. Daniel, 1952.

Vithoulkas, G. *Homoeopathy: medicine of the new man*, Thorsons, 1976.

Useful Addresses

United Kingdom

British Homoeopathic Association
27A Devonshire Street,
London, W1N 1RJ
Tel: 071–935–2163

Hahnemann Society,
Hahnemann House,
2 Powis Place,
Great Ormond Street,
London WC1N 3HT
Tel: 071–837–3297

Society of Homoeopaths
2 Artizan Road,
Northampton NN14HU
Tel: 0604–21400

Institute of Complementary Medicine
Phone between 2–4.30pm.
Tel: 071–237–5165

The Faculty of Homoeopathy
Royal London Homoeopathic
Hospital,
2 Powis Place,
Great Ormond Street,
London WC1N 3HT
Tel: 071–837–2495

The School for Developmental Studies
1 Balfour Road,
Brighton BN1 6NA
Tel: 0273–550540

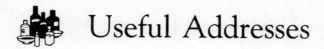

Canada
Canadian Society of Homoeopaths
87 Meadowland Drive West,
Nepean,
Ontario K2G2R9

Australia
Australian Institute of Homoeopathy
21 Bulah Close,
Berdwra Heights,
New South Wales, 2082

USA
American Foundation for Homoeopathy
1508 S. Garfield,
Alhambra,
California CA 91801

William Bergman
Homoeopathic Council for Research & Education
50 Park Avenue,
New York NY 10016
Tel: 212–684–2290

American Institute of Homoeopathy
1585 Glencoe,
Denver CO 80220

New York Homoeopathic Medical Society
110–5671st Avenue 241-H,
Forest Hills,
New York NY 113751

Foundation for Homoeopathic Education and Research
2124 Kitteridge,
Berkeley,
California CA 94704
Tel: 510–649 8930

American Association of Homoeopathic Pharmacies
P.O. Box 2273
Falls Church,
Virginia VA 22042
Tel: 703–532 3237

New Zealand
Gwyneth Gibson
Institute of Classical Homoeopathy
24 West Haven Drive,
Tawa, Wellington,
New Zealand
Tel: 644328051

Courses and Classes

The courses in this list are for those who wish to study homoeopathy in great depth and intend to become practitioners. Most of the courses are of three or four years duration and the majority are part-time (one full weekend per month, several days per week, etc).

The College of Homoeopathy
Regents College,
Inner Circle,
Regents Park,
London NW1 4NS
Tel: 071–487–7416

The London College of Classical Homoeopathy
Morley College,
61 Westminster Bridge Road,
London SE1 7HT
Tel: 071–928–6199

The Midlands College of Homoeopathy
186 Wolverhampton Street,
Dudley DY1 3AD
Tel: 0384–233664

The Northern College of Homoeopathic Medicine
First Floor,
Swinburne House,
Swinburne Street,
Gateshead,
Tyne and Wear NE8 1AX
Tel: 091–4900276

The College of Classical Homoeopathy
Othergates Clinic,
45 Barrington Street,
Tiverton,
Devon EX1 6QP
Tel: 0884–258143

The Scottish College of Homoeopathy
11 Lyndos Place,
Glasgow GA3 3AB
Tel: 041–3323917

Correspondence courses
The School of Homoeopathy,
Yondercott House,
Uffculme,
Devon EX15 3DR
Tel: 0873–856872

Short courses and talks
Many homoeopaths hold classes or give talks for those who wish to learn something of the principles of homoeopathy and perhaps be able to prescribe for first aid and simple ailments in the home. Some of these classes are run by local adult education institutions and others privately. We suggest that you contact your nearest homoeopath and your local adult education institute for up-to-date information about activities in your area.

Pharmacies

If no pharmacy is listed for your area, contact The Homoeopathic Development Foundation or your nearest Citizen's Advice Bureau who should be able to help you locate your nearest supplier.

Avon
Boots the Chemist,
55, Henleaze Road,
Bristol.

Elliots Pharmacy
103 St. Marks Road, Easton,
Bristol 5

Bedfordshire
Kings Wood, Chemist,
25 High Street, Sandy,
Bedfordshire.

Berkshire
F.T. Saunders, Chemist,
41 St. Leonards Road,
Windsor, Berkshire.

Buckinghamshire
Hughes, Chemist,
7 High Street, High Wycombe,
Buckinghamshire.

Channel isles
De Faye, Chemist,
21 David Place, St. Helier,
Jersey.

Learners Chemist,
Temple Court,
St. John,
Jersey.

Cheshire
D.K. Benson, M.P.S.,
6 Grimshaw Lane, Bollington,
Macclesfield.

Cornwall
Peasgood Pharmacy,
1 Market Place, Penzance,
Cornwall.

Cumbria
J.N. Murray, 68 Dalton Road,
Barrow in Furness, Cumbria.

Derbyshire
Eric Dixon, Chemist,
77 Ashbourne Road, Derby.

Weleda (UK) Ltd,
Heanor Road,
Ilkeston.

Devon
Gaynor M. Clark M.P.S.,
70 High Street, Honiton,
Devon.

Dorset
Galen Homoeopathics,
Lewell Mill,
West Stafford,
Dorchester.

Durham
Miller, Chemist,
38 Market Street, Ferryhill,
DL17 8JH.

Essex
Messrs. Rayner,
51 Moulsham Street,
Chelmsford, Essex.

Gloucestershire
James Pharmacy,
19 St. Georges Road,
Cheltenham, GL50 3DT.

Hereford
Chare and Jackson Ltd.,
Broad Street, Hereford,
HR4 9AE.

Hertfordshire
Parry and Jones Ltd.,
61 High Street, Barnet,
Hertfordshire.

Humberside
Priory Pharmacy Ltd.,
148 County Road South, Hull,
Humberside.

Ireland
Rafferty's Pharmacy,
Stillorgan Shopping Centre,
Black Rock,
Co. Dublin.

J.D. McCafferty,
63 Strand Road,
Londonderry.

W.H. Ryan,
32 Strathmillis Park,
Belfast.

Isle of Wight
Small Chemists,
119–120 High Street, Cowes,
Isle of Wight.

Kent
Helios Pharmacy,
J.H. Tomlinson M.P.S.,
92 Camden Road, Tunbridge
Wells, Kent TN1 2QP.

Lancashire
R. and B. Chemists Ltd.,
38 Highbury Road East,
St. Annes-On-Sea, Blackpool.

Leicestershire
Greymarc Ltd.,
19 Prebend Street, Leicester
LE2 0LA.

Lincolnshire
A.W. Mason and Sons,
43 St. Pauls Street, Stamford,
Lincolnshire.

London W.
Ainsworths Pharmacy,
38 New Cavendish Street,
London W1.

A. Nelson and Co. Ltd.,
Homoeopathic Pharmacy,
73 Duke Street, Grosvenor
Square, London W1M 6BY.

London E.
Kingsland Pharmacy,
Kingsland High Street,
London E8.

London EC.
Leon Miller and Co. Ltd.,
9 Tower Hill Place,
London, EC3.

London SW.
Chemco Pharmacy,
268 The Broadway,
Wimbledon,
London SW19.

Sloane, Chemists,
33 Sloane Square,
London
SW1.

London SE.
Warwick Pharmacy,
12 Kingsman Parade,
London SE18.

London N.
Auckland Pharmacy,
27 Ballards Lane, London N3.

London NW.
Martins Chemist,
51 Fairfax Road,
London NW6.

Manchester
Walkden Pharmacy,
4 Hodge Road, Worsley,
Manchester M28 5AT.

Merseyside
Gould Pharmacies Ltd.,
74 Walton Vale, Liverpool 9.

Middlesex
Honeypot Pharmacy,
189 Streatfield Road, Kenton,
Harrow, Middlesex.

West Midlands
Tudor Jones,
1397 Pershore Road, Strichley,
Birmingham 30.

Norfolk
Terence Lincoln, Chemist,
76 Upper St. Giles Street,
Norwich NR2 1LT.

Northamptonshire
E.P. Northover, Chemist,
56 Kingsley Park Terrace,
Northampton.

Northumberland
Bell and Riddle,
Market Place, Hexham.

Nottinghamshire
Gibsons Health Pharmacy,
73 West Gate, Mansfield,
Nottinghamshire.

Oxfordshire
David Morgan, Pharmacy,
11 Besselsleigh Road,
Wootton,
Abingdon OX13 6DN.

Scotland
Freemans Chemist,
7 Eaglesham Road,
Clarkeston,
Glasgow.

Shropshire
J.D. Roche M.P.S., Chemist,
101 Mount Pleasant Road,
Shrewsbury SY1 3EL.

Somerset
G.K. Chemist,
72 Hendford, Yeovil
BA20 1VY.

Staffordshire
Greyfriars Pharmacy,
53 Greyfriars, Stafford.

Suffolk
Anthony Cole, Chemists Ltd.,
46 Hamilton Road, Felixstowe
IP11 7AL.

Surrey
Lindsay Chemist,
181 London Road,
Kingston-Upon-Thames.

Sussex
Astons Chemist,
21 High Street,
Bognor Regis.

Parris and Gearing,
105 Church Road,
Hove.

Cedric Richardson Ltd.,
17 Bishopric, Horsham.

C.H. Roberts,
144 Queens Road,
Hastings.

O.C. Waugh Pharmacy,
Worlds End and Mill Road,
Burgess Hill.

Tyne and Wear
5 Kirkup, 25 West Denton
Park, West Denton,
Newcastle.

Warwickshire
Ivory Chemists,
14 Victoria Terrace,
Leamington Spa,
Warwickshire.

Wiltshire
T.G. Jeary Chemist Ltd.,
13 High Street, Calne
SN11 0BS.

Worcestershire
Boots, Chemists,
72–74 High Street, Worcester.

Yorkshire
Graham Sandell,
20 Hutchliffe Road, Sheffield.

Index

abdomen 61, 63, 65, 67, 70, 72, 73, 75, 78, 79, 81, 83, 85, 87, 89, 91, 93, 97
Anzeiger 4, 5

back, 65, 72, 81, 93
bloodletting 4, 5
Bruckenthal, Baron von 3

cause 17, 18, 38, 41, 43, 45, 50, 51, 110
centesimal scale 11–12
characteristic symptoms 17, 37, 38, 39, 43, 46, 48, 50, 51–2, 54, 59, 60, 64, 67, 68, 74, 78, 84
chest 61, 63, 69, 70, 72, 74, 75, 83, 85, 87, 96, 97
common symptoms 10, 37, 39, 40, 50
contradictions 59
Cullen, Dr 5, 6
cure, 6, 19

decimal scale 12
defence mechanism 22, 23, 26, 30
diet 6, 8, 13
dilution 10
dis-ease 9, 13–15, 18, 20, 26, 30, 31, 36, 46, 55, 107
doses 54, 56, 101, 103
dynamic 12, 14, 21, 23, 24, 26, 31, 34
dynamization 10

ears 75, 78, 83, 89, 90, 96
emotions 8, 10, 84, 85
energy 3, 4, 11, 12, 15, 19, 20, 21, 23, 24, 30, 32, 56
extremities 65, 68, 70, 72, 76, 78, 79, 81, 89, 90, 93
eyes, 51, 52, 61, 63, 67, 68, 71, 72, 77, 79, 80, 81, 85, 90, 96, 100, 103, 104

face 61, 63, 65, 67, 69, 71, 73, 75, 77, 81, 83, 85, 92, 96
female 63, 68, 70, 76, 79, 83, 89, 90, 91
frequency 24, 25, 26, 27

general symptoms 39, 43, 48, 50, 51, 59, 110

Hahnemann, Henrietta 3
Hahnemann, Samuel 2–15, 22
harmony 18, 20, 29, 58
head 38, 40, 42–3, 49, 52–3, 61, 62, 64, 67, 69, 71, 73, 75, 76, 77, 80, 85, 86, 88, 90, 96
health 13–15, 18, 20, 23, 28, 29, 34, 61
health crisis 32–4
health threshold 25
heart 61, 63, 85
Herings law of cure 31

holistic 8, 15, 16, 18, 23, 27, 107, 108

individuality 16, 17, 37
individualize 16, 17, 37, 40, 100

Kent, J.T. 23, 24
Klockenbring 6

Langusius 4
law of similars 6, 9, 11, 17

mental/emotional symptoms 39, 43, 48, 50, 51, 52, 110
metaphysical 6
modalities 40, 43, 46, 48, 50, 61, 63, 66, 68, 70, 72, 74, 76, 78, 79, 82, 84, 85, 87, 89, 91, 93–4, 95, 97
morbific 15, 19
mouth 40, 63, 69, 77, 79, 81, 83, 85, 87, 89, 90, 92, 93, 100, 102

Napoleon 11
neck 40, 65, 79, 80, 81, 85, 93
nose 71, 77, 79, 81, 86, 87, 90, 96

Organon of medicine 7, 14

particular symptoms 39, 40, 43, 50, 52, 110
pattern of existence 25
Peruvian bark 4, 9
potentization 10, 11, 15
potentized 11, 12, 16, 17
Prince Charles 5
provings 10, 16

Quarin, Dr von 3
quinine 5

resonance 23, 25, 26
respiration 63, 65, 74, 87, 90, 93, 95, 96
respiratory 82, 86, 91, 94

Saschen-Gotha, Duke von 6
sensation 40
similar(s) 37, 46, 49, 55
similimum 28, 33
skin 30, 63, 65–6, 68, 70, 72, 76, 79, 83–4, 90, 91, 93, 97
sleep 61, 66, 68, 76, 78, 85, 90
stomach 37, 40, 65, 70, 72, 73, 75, 77, 83, 85, 86, 87, 88, 89, 90, 91, 93, 97
succussion 10
susceptible 22–7, 29, 34, 108
susceptibility 19, 20, 32, 34
symptom picture 9, 10, 36, 37, 38, 39, 46, 49, 58, 59

teeth 61, 75, 76, 77
throat 37, 40, 49, 50, 61, 63, 67, 68, 77, 79, 81, 83, 85, 87, 95, 96
totality 16, 17, 23, 36, 59

urinary 61, 63, 78, 79, 81, 83, 87, 97

vibration 23–5
vibrational frequency 26, 27
vital force 12–15, 18–34

well-being 17, 18, 19, 21, 55, 56